A Twenty Year Fight with Parkinson's Disease

C. Cleveland Piatt

PublishAmerica
Baltimore

First printing

Hardcover 978-1-4489-6465-9
Softcover 978-1-4489-8337-7
PUBLISHED BY PUBLISHAMERICA, LLLP
www.publishamerica.com
Baltimore

Printed in the United States of America

Table of Contents

PRACTICE

It is impossible to know when the writing started
Was it the movement of the pencil or an inspiration?

It is the same story as of the sound
Can it be heard if no one's around?

It seems clear to me and so simple and neat
A car must be put in gear to advance or retreat

Further study indicates that the long journey did not begin with a single step
The way to right a wrong has not been discovered as yet

Is writing really writing if the words do not tell a story
True writing should let the deaf hear and the blind see

Is it the duty of the writer to inform?
Is it lightning and thunder's purpose to announce the storm?

Lightning can strike out of a blue sky
Not all birds of a feather can fly

A TV show can be about nothing
A writer must write about something

An artist is sometimes not an artist until they are dead
A writer is not a writer until they are read

INTRODUCTION

The enclosed is a story of life in Yuma, Arizona, 1934 to 1952; San Diego, California, 1953 to 1958; Los Angeles, California, 1959 to 1960; Santa Barbara, California, 1960 to 1962; Phoenix, Arizona, 1963 to 1986; Lake Wildwood, 1987 to 1995; Mobile, Alabama, 1996 to 1999; Flagstaff, Arizona, 2000 to 2002; Santa Barbara, California, 2002 to 2003. My story must include the fishing and hunting, the fight with cancer, the brain operation and the stories that I must tell to make my story complete.

Vade Long, Jr. was a personal friend for over fifty years. James (Jim) Headington and Herbert (Herb) Lawrence were life-time friends. There are other individuals included in the stories; however the names of those I know are still living have been changed to protect their privacy.

I retired in 1997 to write. I was the senior partner of a CPA firm in Santa Barbara, California. Like many others, I wanted to be a writer. It takes a brave soul to be a writer or a painter. I still work as a matter of necessity, the medical expenses and drug bills are expensive.

I was told that I had Parkinson's disease twenty years ago. The disease is progressive. This book, *A TWENTY-YEAR FIGHT WITH PARKINSON'S DISEASE,* is a realistic story about my struggles in the last twenty years and the struggles of others who have Parkinson's. It is a story of hope and happiness that is lived by us, on life and how most, if given the proper care and knowledge, can lead productive and happy lives for many years. Many doctors are not knowledgeable enough to properly guide a Parkinson's patient, including many of those who are treating themselves.

I lived in Yuma, Arizona, and attended Arizona State University in Phoenix for four years and the University of Arizona, in Tucson, for one year. I was a graduate student at the University of Southern California, Los Angeles, and at San Diego University in San Diego, California. I was a member of the National Honor Fraternity Blue Key, Alpha Tau Omega Fraternity, and Delta Sigma Pi. I was U.S. Treasury agent in Los Angeles and Santa Barbara. I was the Head Resident Auditor of the US DCAA in Santa Barbara, before entering public accounting.

In 1953 and 1954, I was stationed in Europe with the U. S. Army. I love life and writing. I like to travel. I would like to make a speaking tour for the many Parkinson's support groups throughout the United States. It may ease the pain of some sufferers.

March 31, 1999

ROUND ONE

This book is about Parkinson's. The life sentence was handed down, by the neurologist, May 14, 1986. It is about me and must include the story as I lived it. It includes my divorce, and my bout with cancer, as I want you, the reader, to travel with me for twenty years.

It is time to face the music, pay the piper. True teachers will help tell the story. It is a true story.

The simple tests and observations by Dr. Sayer, were duplicated by all the doctors. There are other clues and tests; they add up to an uncontestable fact. I have Parkinson's Disease. I have had 27 neurologists examine me during those twenty years. I have tried all the drugs available for Parkinson's, and I am now considering "deep brain surgery" at the Cleveland Clinic in Ohio. The enclosed copies of correspondence with my doctors tell the story. I am an expert, an intellect, like the neurologist. I test very high on the I. Q. tests. You will travel twenty years with me, suffer and cry. You will find joy and laughter. I will make the trip with you.

We may not have been "aware" of our joint and severable interests, but you will know me body and soul after you read my story. It is important that you know me if you are to appreciate my skills. Get to know my family as you go.

The world is a trying place for a man who has suffered the terror and pains of twenty years as a Parkinson's victim. The leg muscles may lose your walking and standing ability. You could be put on a feeding tube. We are being subjected to terror on a steady, increasing schedule. I would not recommend it to a friend or an enemy. "The Golden Years" have yet to show themselves to me. I would give the next thirty years for ten years "Parkinson Free". We never get better!

In the past twenty years, I have been examined by Neurologists in: Sansom Medical Center, Santa Barbara, California; Veteran's Administration Clinic in Santa Barbara, California; Mayo Brother's Clinic in Phoenix, Arizona; Emory University in Atlanta, Georgia; Veteran's Administration in Flagstaff, Arizona; Cleveland Clinic in Cleveland, Ohio; Ohio State University Hospital in Columbus, Ohio; Veteran's Administration in Columbus, Ohio; Veteran's Administration in Mobile, Alabama; Veteran's Administration in Prescott, Arizona; Veteran's Administration in Los Angeles, California and Veteran's Administration in Fresno, California.

That is enough of the bad sides. The good side has not been discovered yet. Doctors can help ease the suffering by use of drugs and combinations of them. I had a wire inserted in my brain a year ago. It has eased the pain in some areas. Deep brain stimulation is not the answer. It is all we have and is better than doing nothing.

My son worries about his chances. There are no records to show the disease is inherited. The cause is not known. Research dollars are scarce. The available research dollars are increasing and we are making headway.

"Life and love you take."

"Joy and happiness you make."

The attached stories, letters and poems tell a true story.

Today I will try;

Tomorrow I will die

The door to my soul is open; look in. If sad, cry; if happy, smile. Read between the lines — the water is deep. The Jewish say "In a beginning". The Christians say "In the beginning".

MARY JANE HAMILTON

She came into this world on January 19, 1913. She was born Mary Jane Hamilton. She died in 1987 and was buried Mary Jane Hamilton. Most of the time I knew her, she was Mary Jane Piatt. She was not a feminist in any way.

She was born in Tyrone, Pennsylvania and she is buried in Uniontown, Pennsylvania. The Hamilton plot is only a few miles from Tyrone. As a child, her older brother John Hamilton refused to walk with her home from school. He was offended to be with his little sister. He made her walk behind him. She lagged back and when the opportunity presented, ran home. She told her Mother that John had left her. He was given a few pops with the razor strap. Mary Jane laughed, she never had to walk behind him again.

She had been abducted a year before by a mental patient. He carried her into the woods and was caught by her oldest brother, Philip, before he could harm her. He beat the man and took his sister home. She was five or six at the time. She missed the next year of school because of fear.

Her only sister, Nannie, was the oldest of eleven children. She went to school to be a nurse. Times were difficult in the years 1926 — 1929. Mary Jane was needed at home to help with the household duties and the cooking. She was like an indentured slave. Mary Jane hated ironing the sheets and white shirts for her nine brothers and her father.

She showed an interest in sketching and painting in her brief school years. She did not have free time to pursue her interests. Mary

Jane was not abused in modern terms, but her required work was not acceptable. She lept at her first chance to leave. She ran away and was married at sixteen. She was a mother at nineteen.

She found herself keeping house once again, but it was her house and the shirts were always sent out. She missed the finishing a school would have provided. She made up for it by reading everything available. She would stay up all night reading if the book held her interest. The Dale Carnegie Library in Yuma had a good selection of books and she was a regular there.

Mary Jane lived in California from 1924 to 1934. She moved with the family to Yuma, Arizona in 1934. When the first two children were in school, she started to sketch and worked with water colors. She had a keen eye and a remarkable sense of color. She saw things as they were and put the best parts on canvas or paper.

She exhausted the library for books on sketching and painting and started searching elsewhere. She took correspondence courses in related fields. Her early works showed a little promise, but lack of formal training hindered her development.

Arkey Manricks lived next door, a hard working drunk with a body like a Greek god. His wife was a Baptist and very religious. Arkey's uncle lived down the street a half mile and he too was a drunk. Miscarriages and death plagued their life. His wife's Father lived with them. He was blind and hard of hearing and loved the Grand Old Opry show on radio.

Mary Jane had two women friends, Pauline Snow and Sue Hale. She belonged to several different church groups over her life, but did not have a strong feeling for organized religion. She appreciated the fine things money could buy, but money did not mean anything beyond being necessary for providing a good living. She was not greedy. She did like to gamble in Nevada and invested in a rank wildcat operation.

If you are to know me, you must know my Father. He did not walk on water, but I never saw him sink.

OLD IRONSIDE

Lock Albert Piatt, my Father, was born in Conrad, Montana on July 6, 1910
He was the firstborn and was a serious old man beginning to end

He quit school and went to work at the age of seventeen
The family was suffering from a cash shortage, or so it seemed

The big crash of 1929 was the same year my Father was married
Work was where you found it, job to job they harried

Dad found work in California, but during the harvest time in Yuma, Arizona; he loved the work
They worked long hours and the wages were good; he was a packer and a loader

The work lasted a few weeks at a time; you could make three months wages in four weeks
They managed to budget so that they did not panic between valleys and peaks

The packing sheds at peak time, you worked seventy-two hours or more without a break,
when there was work to do

One worker, on a windy day said, "The wind blew, the junk flew and Whitey Ball
took off for an hour or two"

It was hard work, times were tough; Yuma never had a depression
There was work for the hardy; Yuma only suffered a cash recession

He always took the hard jobs, because they paid the highest wages
The crew nicknamed him "Old Ironside"; He never gave up, and was one of the sages

Dad loved the desert, a job offer to work in Yuma, full time; Mom said fine
The wages were not that good; they guaranteed time off and a job during the harvest time

He was twenty-four and known as an old man; he went to work at Arizona Minerals Corporation
Little did he realize that the job would last over thirty years; Yuma said, "Dad was a high spot in creation".

He built a laboratory to study chemistry at home and was soon in charge of the lab
In 1942, he was made the Chief Financial and Operating Officer, while still a young lad

The Arizona Minerals Corporation was way out in the desert when built in 1906, 27th Street today
The Company was bought by the Elgin Water Company, of Illinois; hard cash held sway

Dad was promoted to Vice President of Elgin Corporation and remained the Chief Operation Officer of the Yuma Plant
The Yuma Company was short of cash; they now had extra, a new slant

The Company grew, as Dad had the money to expand; the next ten years, profits were ten times Elgin's investment
He was a good manager, continued his hard working ways, a great accomplishment

We lived on the desert, from home to the office; it was about one mile
The end of my paper boy days and I went to work in the office, the boss's son, the janitor, smile

They paid me $32.00 a month; two or three times a year, a bonus of $100.00. Jackpot!
This job lasted five years and the President of Elgin told Dad to continue to pay me while I was away at ASU. Thanks a lot!

The crew worked most of the time on the many acres of concrete
Joe Tudor was the Foreman and I worked for him four summers; I never accepted defeat

The work was hard labor, shovel and broom time; we were mostly in the sun
In the summer of 1951, we were working in the sun and Yuma had a new heat record, one hundred and twenty one

We loaded trucks and railroad cars, too; like my Father, I enjoyed hard work; it can be fun
My older brother, Dave, Russ Headington, and Tommie Tudor, Joe's son (I lasted four summers), they lasted one

To be fair, they did not have the janitor job, true
I was never without a savings account from my first job, through college, too

My two brothers and I led the good life; like Dad, we all loved Yuma, winters and summers, too

Dad's perks included cars, country clubs, the Arizona Club, unlimited expense account, and the airplane he flew

He continued to manage the company until it closed in the early sixties; he was fraught
The acres and acres of concrete, near the hospital and 27th Street, may still mark the spot

Yuma was always home and Dad was known to say
When God made the Yuma desert, He made it His way

My Mother, weeks before she too, left the world we know and my lights were again dim
Said that Dad "Was the kindest and best man she ever met and that I was JUST LIKE HIM"
August 13, 1998

MY EARLY LIFE, BEFORE PARKINSON'S

Life was much simpler when we grew up. There were not near as many no's in those days.

GROW UP TIME

Mother was born on the nineteenth of January in 1913
Chestnut brown were her eyes and hair of the same sheen

Fair to look at and beautiful to see
Five older and four younger brothers, she was a Queen Bee

Her Mother, Laura Catherine "Katie" Thompson Hamilton was heavy and not very tall
Mary Jane Hamilton was five foot three inches and two inches taller

Grandmother Katie was from the old school ways
Housework and cooking filled all her days

She must have saved the energy needed for she succeeded
In having eleven children, some assistance is dearly needed

John Hayes Hamilton, Grandpa, was a big man - six foot, two inches and two hundred twenty pounds
His hair was gray and his eyes brown, serious by nature, he often frowned

Grandpa Hamilton went to work in the Pennsylvania Coal Mines when he was nine
He drank like a gentleman, always sober; he started chewing Beechnut Tobacco at the same time

When he married Katie, he was foreman of a lumber mill
In Tyrone, Pennsylvania. They lived there twenty years without many frills

California called and the Hamilton family moved there in 1924
El Centro was their first stop and in 1928, they said nevermore

Pennsylvania summers are hot, but not like El Centro where it is hot, hot, hot
They moved to Salinas, California, where the weather is mild and hot is not

Grandmother Katie was a great cook and kept a home well readied up
Mary Jane spent her days cooking and ironing until she was grown up

She ironed white shirts for the men and sheets for the bed
The whole family worked and Mary Jane overworked, but well fed

Took the first boat out as the saying goes, flew the coop
She married my Father Lock Albert Piatt in 1929

My Father was born July 6, 1910 in Conrad, Montana
The oldest of a family of five, three brothers, one sister and he

His Father, Grandpa Paul C. Piatt was born on May 7, 1887 in Devils Gate, North Dakota
He was a farmer, railroad man, a worker who also drank and partied

Grandmother Maude Cleveland Piatt was born in Carolltown, Minnesota in 1878
She was a teacher; one brother was a doctor and one a lawyer, refined and a lady

She was special to me; she always sent me $10.00 when she wrote to me
While in the Army in Germany, a letter from home was great, the money free

Grandmother Maude was always interested in what I did or so it seemed
She did not like my Mother a bit; my Mother treated her with respect and inwardly steamed

Grandpa Paul C.'s Father was C. C. Piatt, a farmer in Cooperstown, North Dakota
He was an Indian Scout with Colonel Forsyth's Scouts who won the battle with Chief Roman Nose, September 17, 1868

The Battle of Beecher Island, Arickaree Fork of the Republican River, in Colorado where the scouts won
Fifty-two scouts against over three hundred Indians, fifteen scouts were wounded, five died, fifty-two Indians dead, no fun

JIM AND IKE

Ike was born in California, Jim and Ike were buddies before they could talk
Jim was born in Yuma, Arizona, down the block and it was a very short walk

They lived in the country across the street and down the road from a pig farm
There were also horses, cattle, chickens, goats, sheep and rabbits to charm

But the best thing of all was a multitude of canals and irrigation ditches that meandered throughout the valley
The people that lived in the valley were not wealthy by any tally

We both were born during the great depression
In Yuma, a farm town, it was little more than a cash recession

We had plenty to eat — meat, vegetables and fish we caught
Hard cash was hard to find, but we suffered naught

Jim was five and I was six when we learned to swim in the canal
Summers were just great in Yuma, 110 degrees is fine for swimming, well?

When you are five and six, great play days are hot or cold
Once we showed that we could swim and take care of each other, we were free and bold

A year later when I was seven and a half and Jim was almost seven too
We planned each day's adventure, told our Mom's where we were going and what we planned to do

We left in the mornings early and told our parents we would be back at four
Our allowed territory covered about one and a half miles door to door

They asked about lunch and many times we told of our plans that were flexible
There was a different menu for the whole summer; everything the farmers and ranchers grew was edible

This was a place where plums, crab apples, figs and apricots grew
Down the road was a ranch with pomegranates, too good to be true

They were big, red, tart and lasted all summer, next was a pecan orchard waiting
Next door to the pecans was a watermelon patch for the taking

Down the main canal, a half mile, was a farmer who grew grapes
There was a strawberry patch across the canal at the Head Gates

The area we roamed was a small community and the kids were few
The many summers, we knew the farmers and they knew who the kids were too

We never had a written or oral contract either, but no one complained, ever
I think about it today in wonder, the melon patch was not harvested, ever

The nut trees were never fully harvested, neither the pomegranates nor the grapes, why?
Times were bad and cash was scarce, but none of us went hungry in the valley, we caught fish to fry

We took care to never damage a crop, took only what was lunch
I doubt if any of our benefactors are alive today, but thanks a bunch

The road to the main canal was partially paved, the asphalt turned soft in spots, when it was hot
We ran the half-mile up Avenue C to the bridge, which was our main swimming spot

The bridge was eight feet above the road and four feet above the water, twelve feet from the water to the top
We thought we were brave when we learned to dive off the fourth step, a pretty far flop

A couple of years later, I dove off the scary, high-up top
I don't remember my dive, but Jim's, a little later, was a flop

From the bridge, another half mile, was the Head Gates and Cooper Ditch, too
This was our second favorite swimming spot and our best fishing hole, when there was nothing else to do

We always had one little line and fishhooks and we could make a pole
There were blue gills, a few bass and carp; Jim's Dad loved the blue gills from the hole

Sometimes we would go the extra mile to Ruby's corner store at lunchtime
This swimming hole had a nifty rope to swing on and we had lunch for a dime

A dime would buy a large milk and apple pie
A penny bought you a Baby Ruth, too — sigh!

In the next few years, we learned a few tricks, as well
The rope was tied thirty feet up in a tree; it was swell

People shopping for groceries would sometimes watch us play
We showed off some, did our best tricks and had fun each day

Time to head home was a quarter to two
Happy and smiling, homeward we flew

It was one half mile to Cooper Ditch and one half mile to the bridge on Avenue C
We swam and floated to Cooper Ditch, over the Gates, and on to the bridge, happy and free

It was now two-thirty and time to run the half-mile home
We always made it home by three and never went alone

Jim and Ike loved the valley, with so many things to do
They lived there for eleven years, many excursions and time flew

They are alive today, though getting old
They have many stories, yet to be told

CRAWDAD FISHING WITH IKE AND JIM

Maybe we dreamed it, someone may have told us, but one day we knew how to catch crawdads or crayfish
We were five and six, in the woods behind our lot was a small irrigation ditch, it was part of our wish

There were not many things that we needed, or wanted, on this day
The long hot days of summer were our greatest treasures, time to play

We seldom wore shoes and cut off Levis have pockets and make a good swimming suit
T-shirts are all we needed for our formal wear to be complete, who cared a hoot

This day it was one hundred and twelve degrees in the shade
Yuma Valley is the greatest place in the whole world; summertime and we had it made

The water was two to three feet deep and there were many small pools as well.
We swam in the pools and splashed up and down the ditch; it was swell

There was the occasional snake, a frog now and then, but always in summer there were crawdads to catch
We caught polliwogs, watched them grow legs, lose their tails and turn into frogs

Crawdads, when they are very small, are translucent pale green
As they grow up they turn a dark green, as they grow old they get mean

The biggest ones add a bright red and deep purple to their shell
Their claws are a dark red and are scary and vicious as well

They use their claws for fighting and grab a finger or two if you are not careful
We were tough, if they got a hold of one of us, we did not cry, but were often tearful

The past two years we had studied the crawdads life pattern and style, we knew no fear
The ditch was dry for a day once or twice each month and they seemed to disappear

They were still in the pools, as they never went dry
Part of our daily adventures, was to learn something new, we would at least try

It did not take that much time, but it took a heap of raw nerve, we located their holes
It seems they were very good tunnel makers, almost as good as the moles

The holes were full of muddy water; the only way to find out what made the holes was a tough test
I don't remember who the first to discover it was, but when you put your hand in, they did the rest

They would grab your finger with one or two claws; you pull them out real slow
When it was a big one, red and purple and huge red claws, they would not let go

You were not allowed to cry no matter how hard they pinched, but you could yell
They sometimes hurt a bunch, when you had to yank them off, if you cried a little, no one would tell

We could catch a few crawdads when the ditch was dry
The good fishing was in the pools where you never had to cry

In Yuma, Arizona not many people knew how good they were to eat
In New Orleans, my wife loved them and now considers them a great treat

The restaurant was at Jack's Brewery and my wife and I were there for lunch
The southern gentleman next to us was eating crawdads; they were on a tray, 50 to 60 of them, a bunch

He broke the tails, from the heads and bodies, with a shove, and a bite, the tail was gone
The juice dripped down his chin, a grin on his face, the pile disappeared and it did not take long

It seems that the deep-south people have known for a long time about crayfish
They have barbeque parties where crawdads were the featured main dish

This day we were after crawdads and each had the necessary supplies

Six foot of line, a few small pieces of gunnysack and also of bacon rind, no flies

It had been said that big time, city folks, used flies for fishing
We used sow bugs for bait when fishing for bluegill or perch and dough ball for catfish

We cut an arrow weed pole about four feet long, tied the line and it worked just fine
On the other end of the line we tied either the little pieces of gunnysack or bacon rind

We had been explorers for two or three years by the time we were five or six
If we gave a yell, someone came running, never tested it, we never got in a fix

The deeper pools were best; we dropped our line in the big pool, it was time for the show
In minutes, we both felt a tug, they chew on the bait for a while and you pull them in real slow

They grab with both claws and don't like to let go
Slowly you pull them up the bank then pop them into the bucket

The few smart ones let go before they are pulled out of the pool
Some let go on land and you scoop them up, but you have to play cool

In the water, they swim backwards and are awful fast, on land they crawl slow
You pick them up behind their claws; they can pinch pretty good, as we now know

Our parents tell us that it is hot and we should play inside until late afternoon

We know that every day we can, we must explore our world, for we grow up too soon

It was lunchtime, the bucket was full; we were close to home
We were not expected to come home for lunch, were always welcomed and we did not lunch alone

The summers in Yuma were to grownups terribly hot
Summers were the best time of year and to us hot it was not

Mrs. Stillwater, our first grade teacher, lived next to the bridge, our favorite swimming hole
Sometimes she would invite us to have lunch with her; she was a famous writer and a dear soul

That is another story, maybe many more, for she was very kind to us, and an explorer as well
Summers, in Yuma, were very special and important to us; we have much to tell

MRS. STILLWATER

Mrs. Stillwater was a very special teacher, who I met my first day of school
She taught the first grade, Crane School, in the Yuma Valley, as kids say today, she was cool

She was a widow, lived alone on Avenue C, next to the Canal Bridge, where Jim and Ike swam
Mrs. Stillwater was a famous writer of children's stories; I will always be a fan

She taught first grade for many years, because she loved the kids, the old timers and the newcomers
We had a candy sale in the first grade; she said, "Ikey, you make change, because you are so good with numbers"

That simple compliment probably made me what I am today
She encouraged everyone; she always had a kind word to say

We passed her home on the way to our favorite swimming spot
It was normal to slow down as you passed, we liked her a lot

The thought of fresh baked cookies and a cool drink, often entered our minds
In summers, she quite often would be waiting for us, so it seemed, she was kind

We never went so far as to yell or go whistling by
Nor did we try to hide, with practice, we learned to appear shy

It was so easy for us to tell, she knew our motives better than we did
But it was like a poker game, you may bluff, it is not a fib

On special occasions, special to us anyway, she might ask us to come back for lunch
We had been warned many times to be leery of strangers, our mothers approved of Mrs. Stillwater, thanks a bunch

She took an interest in all our travels and expeditions too
We blabbed a book full, maybe two, before lunch was through

I look back in amazement, two barefoot boys, with cut off Levi's and a white t-shirt
Acting like grown up explorers, good table manners, and we did flirt

The many years we knew her, she was always dressed up, like on the center stage
She was always prim and proper; would laugh when we told a whopper and was a sage

Years later, when I moved away, Mrs. Stillwater had invited us to lunch to say goodbye
I can't be sure, but when we thanked her and said goodbye, she had a tear in her eye

She will always be with us, her kindness and guidance, and the time she shared
A special teacher, one who loved to work with kids, and one who cared

MURDER ONE

The man had a machete and he rubbed the edge over the covers on the bed.
I was terrified, why was he here, why did he want to kill me, a small cut and I bled

The month was July and the covers were not much of a shield against the machete
Fear was deep and I could not move, could I be a coward afraid of what I could not see

Someone stirred in the next room, the machete was lifted from my leg, the villain lingered
I laid still, afraid to move, my eyes were wide open, but still I could not lift a finger

July in Yuma, Arizona is hot, air conditioning we had not
My sixth birthday starting off with a killer's visit, I was distraught

Thirty minutes passed or was it thirty hours; I was dripping with sweat
Dad's voice penetrated the darkness, with a good morning, I got up; did I tell him, I'm thirty and not yet.

THE HEADINGTONS

(as I saw them)

The earliest picture I have of Mr. Headington, is on a milking stool
He was very friendly and nice, but don't call anyone in his family a fool

In 1940, we started buying milk from his one cow Dairy
Mr. Headington worked for the Telegraph Co., sold real estate, and treated everyone fairly

He always said he raised me, and in part, it is true
I spent so much time there; I was part of the crew

Mrs. Headington, I still see in the kitchen baking, cooking and cleaning
She was a beautiful person, strong, wise and fair, not one for dreaming

She was always especially nice to me
She often told Jim she wished he was more like Ikey

One day, Ike threw the football, broke the window, Jim had a fit
Jim laughed, smiled and yelled, "Ikey broke it, Ikey broke it!"

The youngest of five children was Gerry or Butch, AKA the little brother of Russ
He spent a lot of time with Ike and Jim; was a good friend to both of us

Louise had two older, and two younger brothers, all misters
She was pretty, intelligent and sweet, but she should have had a sister

Gus was the oldest, the leader, a very good athlete and a scholar
When Jim and I needed help, it was for Russ we hollered

Bill, the 2nd oldest, was forever playing tricks on Jim and Ike
He was a good boxer, they all were, and when asked to put on the gloves with him, we would take a hike

We often helped Mrs. Headington in the churning of butter and the cranking of the ice cream maker
Cookies, cake and pastries were always a reward or a bribe — she was a great baker

Prayer and church were required, a regular part of the family routine
Mr. Headington did not curse, did not drink, but in church was seldom seen

Jim, Gerry and Ike played together for as long as their memories serve them
Jim and Ike never considered it a responsibility, we didn't take care of Gerry; he was part of the group

Jim and Gerry sometimes had contests, to see who could put the most pepper on the breakfast eggs, no salt
The eggs would be black; completely covered with pepper, I would default

Mrs. Headington fixed Mr. Headington a baked pig's head; he loved it, cheers
The apple in the mouth, the pig smiling; he was especially fond of the ears

Mr. Headington also liked the perch we three caught at Coopers Ditch, in the spring and fall
Mrs. Headington would fry them crisp and he ate them, bones and all

Mr. Headington was a stout man, who enjoyed his food; I don't remember anything he did not like
They all had good appetites, Mrs. Headington always cooked extra and she always set a place for Ike

Russ, Bill and Louise were never around much, we had the place to enjoy
We had very few chores to do, if any, mostly we explored the valley

The Crane School sponsored a Boy Scout Troop; it was a study and fun-time group
The troop put on an annual fund raising carnival; we always needed money in the troop

Russ was the best boxer in the valley and they had trouble finding someone to box with him
The last year Russ was there, he was listed as the Masked Marvel; Bill had a plan to win

Everyone knew who the Masked Marvel was; Bill was willing to give him a fight
Round one, they exchanged a few punches, to find out what it is about; then Bill got it right

Bill hit Russ's mask around so Russ could not see
Then Bill would pound him, hit him hard and often, sting like a Bee

It seemed that it was a one sided fight against the man who could not see

The next round it started as before, but Russ had changed plans, took off his mask, it was meant to be

The last round Russ pounded Bill, he hit hard and often. Bill gave a good accounting of himself
Russ was too skilled and tough for the rest of the valley would be tough; he deserves the championship trophy on his shelf

Jim and Ike were best friends, that is until fight time at the Yuma Carnival Corral
No cut off Levi's for this fight night; trunks are worn by the boxers, boxers have no best pal

The bell sounds round one, the two former pals rush to the center of the ring
They throw lefts, rights, uppercuts, round houses and jabs, the gloves would sing

Round two was more of the same, this was no game, this was war; you do your best to rack up a score
The crowd was happy to see the spirited fight, we were knocked down, tripped and fell, they would roar

Round three and the crowd still wanted more blood and we did our best to comply
We didn't throw as many punches as in round one, but not many less, our eyes were dry

The fight was long and fought toe to toe; the rest was up to the judges
Fight one the judges said, was a draw; we gave it our best and held no grudges

The next year they asked me to fight Jim again; no one wanted to fight the Headington boys

Ike agreed to one more try, Jim was a good boxer and fighting him was not one of life's joys

Year two was a lot like year one; we were boxers out to win a fight when the bell rang
We pleased the crowd again, gave them more of the same, we threw a lot of punches, our gloves sang

Round three, bruised, bloodied, and sore, we awaited the judges' final score
The crowd enjoyed the fight and applauded the decision; the match was a draw once more

Another year and fight time again, Jim was improved, but no one wanted to fight him
They decided that six of us should fight a free for all, you're out if you are knocked down, sink or swim

The bell rang and Jim charged out, knocked one guy down and charged another fighter, not me
I exchanged a few punches, but played it cool; I anticipated a battle with Jim in round three

Jim was throwing punches in frenzy; knocked down the second boxer, it was still round one
I continued to throw a few punches, basically for warming up; Jim was saving me for last and fun

I was going to be as fresh as possible, so I conserved my energy for Jim
Jim charged the third boxer like a bull, the boxer drew back and Jim fell over his leg, a sin

The Judge threw Jim out and it was my turn to smile, Jim called for a whistle, said he was tripped

It was a bad break, but Jim had tried and it is one of those things, he flipped

I disposed of one and there were two of us left, we pounded each other, I looked for a slip or a flaw
We traded punches the next round, neither was able to knock the other down, the fight was declared a draw

That third year was my last; I retired from the ring undefeated
I never asked Jim, but I am sure he felt like he was cheated

Mr. Headington, was used by Ike, for a reference, every time he needed one
Ike went to work after college, The United States Treasury Department, his day in the sun

The FBI sent investigators to interview Mr. Headington, and didn't tell him why
He thought Ike was in trouble, and Mr. Headington told Ike later, that the FBI almost made him cry

Three years later, the FBI was back to see Mr. Headington again, this time Mr. Headington was tough
Why were they asking about Ike? They acted tough and he treated the FBI rough

The FBI decided to be nice and told Mr. Headington that I had applied for a secret Government Clearance
Ike was not in trouble and the Government Agents gave him their assurance

Mr. and Mrs. Headington were special people, living in Yuma Valley, at a special time
They have moved to greener pastures, Louise moved, Russ, Bill, Jim and Gerry are in Yuma doing fine

The Luckys are or were friends of mine, part of my growing up.

LUCKY'S CASINO

R. H. Lucky was a grand old man; Yuma, Arizona was his town
Ike was his newspaper delivery boy in 1945 and Mr. Lucky never let Ike down

Ike's route covered the downtown area, typically called Main Street
J. C. Penney, Sears, The Imperial Hardware Store, Vade's Clothing Store were a small part of Ike's beat

Sanganetti's Department Store and a little later, King's Men's Store
The downtown stores were the main shopping places in the county for rich and poor

There were three movie shows on Main Street; the Yuma was the best
The Lyric and Orphan were the others, but their names put Ike's memory to the test

The Post Office building was next to J. Cash Penney's Store
The Immaculate Conception Church was across the street; it burned and is no more

This area was called South Main; it follows that the other was North Main
North Main had a watering hole or two, a bum or three, a house and was off limits to the tame

Yuma had two hotels downtown; the old one was the Arizona and had a pleasant dining room
It was near the Yuma Southern Pacific Railroad Depot and one could hear the trains puff and boom

Two drug stores, with soda fountains, and a super banana split
One had booths and it was there that the teenagers liked to sit

North of town, on the Colorado River, sat the infamous Yuma Territorial Prison
The walls were five feet thick and it was hot during the spring and summer season

The cells were small, little ventilation, built to punish the meanest, hardened criminals, and they were hot, hot, hot
Yuma was a crossing point to California and was a famous western town where horse thieves were shot

From the time Ike can remember and it is still true today, Ike loves old Main
Mr. Lucky was a kind and generous man, fair to all and never vain

Every month we collected for the Yuma Daily Sun
Penney and Sears never tipped; Mr. Lucky always gave one

A warm smile, a pleasant greeting, and extra twenty-five cents
It bought a hamburger and a coke; Ike forgave the other skinflints

This is about the Lucky casino, where the elite meet
You need to know a bit more about Mr. Lucky, life on the street

Summer time it was hot on Main Street, Hot days were 110 degrees or more
The street was hotter, stores were cold; delivering papers was a chore

The local house on Ike's route, Ike delivered the paper up stairs in the back room
The Lady in charge was very nice, left a fifty-cent tip; Ike hummed a happy tune

In his early days, Mr. Lucky opened the "Sweet Shop" across from Yuma High
It was a famous spot for lunch or to meet after school to say Hi!

Mr. Lucky ran for Justice of the Peace in Yuma and won
He served for many years and opened the Gretna Green Wedding Chapel before he was done

Ike remembers the Casino as he played dominoes and shot pool there in days long ago
There were a number of other investments by Mr. R. H. Lucky; about them you should know

He invested in a Taxi Company, a Bus Company, a Drag Line Company and the Casino Pool Hall
Mr. Lucky was a hard worker and firm believer in the future of Old Yuma, not a fancy new mall

The Casino is the oldest operating pool hall in Arizona and an "In place" for fun
They do a great business — restaurant, bar and the poolroom, now managed by Bob, Mr. Lucky's son

The old town was boarded up a few years ago; the Lucky's family and a few others stayed to fight
The new malls took over; the closed stores were a terrible sight

Young Lucky believed in Yuma and knew that things would change in time

It was a long fight, but things changed, stores reopened and the Casino is doing fine

The Casino, where the elite meet
To visit, to play, to drink and eat

FISHERMEN THREE

In Yuma, Arizona, we started the Yuma High Fishing Club in the year 1951
Vade, Herb, and Ike and a few, well-chosen classmates, joined for fun

But it was the three of us who fished and did some hunting, too
In time, we knew the Colorado River, lakes and every slew, where fish swam and birds flew

High school, we passed our classes, but we never wasted time
We did not waste our adventure time doing homework assigned

With our Huckleberry Finn garb and our classic fishing gear
We waded in the lakes all summer, fall, winter, and spring without fear

Be the weather cold or hot, we gave the fish a challenge and made the California fishermen sour
Fishermen came in airplanes, expensive boats they rented, fishing guides by the hour

Sunday afternoon, as we prepared to go home, we loved going to the fishing camp to show our
catch
Our catch was super, they would be surprised and the amazed, which made us feel rich

We were three not-rich boys who knew the lakes and how to fish
Plush boats and guides were not in our budget or for which we did not wish

Our car was a 1939 Pontiac Fire Chief; we used to floorboard the car to climb the desert hills
We camped out on the ground with the rattlesnakes and rocks, old bleached out Levi's, a white shirt and no frills

We fished together for three summers; we did some hunting too
Ducks, geese, dove, deer, quail and rabbits, they both ran and flew

We never missed a school dance, play, or the Junior or Senior Prom — we had a ball
We attended all football, basketball, baseball, and track meet games — happy times all

Herb and Ike's steady girls slowed the adventures a little
Vade played the field and was a grasshopper who did not play the fiddle

Herb took leave of us early, too early in life, he did not say goodbye
We called Herb one night, years ago and they said he had passed away last week, I did cry

The sun shines bright on the memory of those days of us three
We were part of the land, young, in good health and free

Since then forty-seven winters have come and gone away to fast
We all three had sons who we raised in years past

Yes, Herb moved on to greener pastures a long time ago, we miss him still today

The two fisherman are now suffering the path age leads and turning
gray

The three fishermen are now two and will too soon be one and none
Herb, Vade and Ike have but few regrets, we lived and had some fun

The beautiful Colorado River we knew was a half-mile wide and swift
Today you can walk across, we used to swim; times change if you get
my drift

August 1, 1998

HE PULLED A GUN

One never knows what can happen when you are having fun, sometimes acting the fool
Gil and I have been good friends since we were in high school

He went directly into the Navy; he served for four years, mostly at sea
I was drafted out of college and spent two years in the Army, mostly in Germany

He belonged to the same Fraternity; we were roommates, not like the odd couple, we were both neat
We did not want to live in the fraternity house; too much confusion to study, too much social heat

We rented a four-room apartment located in the backyard of our landlord
He treated us as adults; we had company, but never a loud party. It was great and one we could afford

We both had the GI Bill; we also received help from home; a little more came my way
We both worked part time, Gil more than me; at one time I was his assistant bus driver, those kids made my day

We were serious students with a goal; time was to us a treasure
The main reason we lived off campus, freedom to study quietly at our leisure

We still managed to go to the fraternity parties, dances, sings, and sporting events; everything there was to see
But our main goal was to earn a college degree, find a future and seek immortality

The place was kept clean and neat; we were never afraid to bring friends by
There was never an argument; we each did or seemed to do his share, no cause to cry

Mother had given me a nine inch black and white TV; it was great, we sometimes took a break and caught the Tuesday night fight
Our favorite show was Maverick; we always had four or five couples to watch it on Sunday night

It was a date that fit our budget and we really had a good time; we served soda, beer, and snacks as we could
The girls always enjoyed a short break from Sunday studies and the TV, little as it was; our eyes were good

The fraternities still did a little hazing in those days; our group was very mild
They did drop Vade and I off in the desert, ten or fifteen miles from Tempe, we acted wild

Gil was a few years older than most of the fraternity guys and didn't want us old vets to get hurt
He came back and picked us up as soon as he could get away; we walked three miles and ate a little dirt

We three played along with the group and never let them know about the ride
We took our fraternity serious, were all very active, this event set aside

Mike and I were serious poker players and would sometimes have a game
We had six or seven regular players and usually a drop in or two, they were all sane

That is except for one, uninvited, unwanted, feared and he did not play with a full deck
The other six players did not want to play, they folded; I was the only player to check

My cards were running good that Sunday afternoon, I decided on the spot to call, without seeing a card
Gil was being bluffed by a couple of goons, I naturally took Gil's side; they were in the yard

Gil had a telephone call a few minutes earlier; he had to go pick up two sorority girls who needed a ride
They were pledges, who were being hazed, by the sorority, dropped at a service station, on the roadside

He had been gone for thirty minutes when we heard two cars slide to a stop in our driveway
The two girls came running in the apartment and yelled that there was going to be a fight, not if I had my say

Gil was outside alone; I jumped up and ran out the door, without a second thought
I, of course, expected the other players to join me; that was without being sought

One of the players was a 265-pound star football player; I wanted him on my side
There was a tree just in front of the door and as I rushed out, I saw the guy pull a gun

I froze, was not seen, stepped back inside, told the players they had a gun, to call the police
There was no decision to be made, Gil was my friend; I stepped out and past the tree

It was years ago, but as I recall, it was only a brief period before the problem was solved
The guy with the gun told me there was going to be a fight; I told him that if there had to be a fight, make it a fair one

I was going to stall for time as long as it was possible
Gil was standing beside his car, about twenty feet from the guy with the gun

When I came out, I stopped about six feet from the gunman; Gil and the other mug were still in the driveway
It is strange how so many things can pass through one's mind; under the circumstance, the memory is crystal clear to this day

I looked across at Gil; he was covered with perspiration, but was outwardly calm
The guy with the gun didn't look that tough; I thought of taking him out, he should have been home with his mom

If I was forced to make a play, I should be a little closer to the Joker with the gun
It was only a short time and I was a foot closer to him; he didn't act drunk, they thought they were having fun

It was not entirely new to me, being under pressure, and facing trouble; someone is looking after me
There was no way that I could leave Gil out their facing those thugs alone. Do what you can and see what is to be

The girls he had rescued, the thugs were trying to pick them up in Scottsdale, where they had been dropped
They had tried to force Gil to stop, had chased him home, eighty-five miles an hour at times

Without the gun, it would have been a laugh; the gun took all the laughter out of it
We were both Veterans of Foreign Wars, liked out life; did not want to leave it while still young and fit

We continued to talk; I was ready to make a move if necessary, not unless I had to, not wanting to play the fool
Gil must have known I was stalling as best I could; he was calm and looking back, it amazes me, but I was cool

The Army trained me to be a killer; they told me to run when you are out gunned, fighting is no fun
Fight a man with a knife only when you are cornered, run if you can, it was late to run

I was prepared to take him, but only if there was no other way
The man was ever so proud of the gun, and his friend didn't have very much to say

All of my what- ifs ended with a flying tackle; the gunman was on the ground face down, without his toy
There was no warning, a flash of light so fast, if you have not been watching close; you would have missed it, pure joy

Gil and I had a good day before the thug's visit, sweated out a poor hand, enjoyed a late supper
Thanks go to our next invited guest, the last to arrive that night; he was the party upper

There was no sound that I heard, no tires squealing, no siren; no policeman yelling
The officer came around the corner of the front house on the fly; the officer was working, a story worth telling

He never drew his revolver, never said hi; he flat tackled that man on the fly
My parents had always told me, the police have a difficult job to do; tonight was why

The police paddy wagon pulled up the drive, took the girls and my friend to jail
Let them go after they signed a complaint, put the thugs in jail, they spent the night and posted bail

We found out later from the police report, the thugs were freshman college students, out for a laugh, no sale
The gunman now has a felony record, he pleaded guilty to a concealed gun charge, sentenced to six months in jail

They did not get a laugh, we found no amusement, did not enjoy the show, had no fun
The other poker players, we found out that night, would give up the game at the sight of a gun

The strangest thing, besides a guy hiding under the bed, was that the gun was not loaded; the thug ran a bluff
The gunman was lucky; there was my shotgun, the thought flashed before me when I first saw the gun, enough

Gil and I graduated from college and spent our last summer in Aqua Caliente, working in a cantaloupe shed
We worked hard, it was in the Arizona desert, it was hot, it was educational, the pay was good and we were fed

It was my last job that required hard labor; Gil was in charge of the record keeping so he did not work as hard
My last night I was pushing a truck, with five or six crates on it, it was tough work

Up and down the dock, up the ramp, into the truck, each trip felt like it was my last; it was, thank the Lord
Gil didn't think I would make it through the night, took my truck and gave me his clipboard

Without his help, I would not have finished that night; I made $90 for that last night
I had a job offer in Los Angeles, Arthur Anderson, a National CPA Firm, offered me $440, a month, $20 a day, right?

The shed was closing down, this was the last week; I quit that night, my last real labor
Gil stayed to close the shed; he was an executive with a clipboard, not a real officer with a saber

Gil and I took a trip to California looking for a position; a job for the future was what we sought
We stopped in Riverside where Gil interviewed for a position with an electronics firm; a wife and a job he got

He retired from the same firm this summer, forty-years later; time to play
He married the receptionist there; the same one I had met that first day

The honor was mine; I was best man, when they were married in Riverside
If ever life brings me more trouble than I can abide, I would like a friend like Gil at my side

We have met a few times over the past forty years, raised our children, had our careers
Gil was a very successful executive; I know he should have been the president, if the founder and owner had not been. Cheers!

We still talk on the phone once in a while; Gil is in my thoughts and is a good friend
With all the nuts in the world this day, the man with a gun, before the start, could have been the end

September 10, 1998

I AM A MAN

I am a man, any man that you may meet.
I live in the same town, on the same street.
Why don't you accept me for what I am?
I am a man; I live, breathe, have feelings the same as you.
I am capable of love, work and as a friend I can be true.
I try to buy a home in the nice part of town.
The house is for sale; the owner turns me down.
Why don't you accept me for what I am?
We worship God; I worship the same God as you.
Maybe not in the same way, but with the same feelings as you do.
In this life I can't live with you on the same plain.
In the hereafter you and I will be the same.
Why don't you accept me for what I am?
It is true I won't eat of the swine.
Your skin has a different look than mine.
I live, love, breathe, eat, yearn and I am a man.
Why don't you accept me for what I am?

1955 or 1956

English Lit Class, Arizona State University, Phoenix, Arizona

The professor wrote the following on this paper. "Anyone writes this strongly should write more." He put the poem up on the screen and the class discussed it for half the period.

THE BIG SECRET

The family had planned for a big party, in secret, for the past eight years.
Not one of his three children dreamed that it would actually happen, no way and no fears.

No male member of Thompson's family had lived past sixty, in two hundred and twenty years; the last died in 1979, at sixty-three.
Thom, as he was called, and his wife, Mary Jane, who always said, he would live to be a hundred and three.

They had married when they were eighteen years old, their parents did not approve.
The oldest child, Thompson Jr., was born five months later; he had nothing to prove.

It was said, "He was premature and overweight, because of a glandular problem." Sigh!
He weighed ten pounds and five ounces and came into the world with a hardy cry.

Thompson was at his dad's urging an attorney, who specialized in palimony.
He considered his father a boar and a party would be a waste of time; he went along with the planning baloney

He could promise anything; his dad was a dead duck and would be lucky to reach fifty-eight.
His dad was plain old white trash from Mobile, Alabama, a third generation fry cook, fifty pounds overweight

Mary Jane in twelve months gave birth to their second child; Peggy Sue was carried nine months and a day
Peggy Sue, no glandular problem, weighed seven pounds and nine ounces; her cry held the hounds at bay

Peggy Sue considers her Father a no good, loud, dirty, uneducated slob and a smarty.
For years, she has led the party planners for her father's all family birthday party.

Peggy Sue was expelled from school in the ninth grade; she had a child born with a glandular problem, too.
Hector Thompson Hendricks, eight pounds, fourteen ounces, born four months premature; it is true.

Twelve months later, Hector had a little brother born with a happy smile and a black mane.
Granville Thompson Hendricks, a boy, seven pounds, ten ounces, and called Thom by Mary Jane.

Eleven months later Thompson's third child was born, full term and eight pounds.
Robert Lee was the Sheriff when he grew up and his dad was proud to go with him on his rounds.

Robert Lee married his high school sweetheart when she graduated a year after Robert Lee.
They do not have any children yet, but are both capable and the doctor said, "Wait and see".

Robert lee does not care about the party, hopes his dad lives that long and his mother gets the brass ring.
He thinks his dad is a hard-headed, hard-working cuss, who is fair but rules the family like he was king.

Thompson was a fry cook when he got married. He worked double shifts to get by and he was a Shriner
He was a dreamer who on a rare day off had a beer too many and stopped for ribs at a small diner.

Jim Bob offered Thompson a beer; they started talking about cooking, the roll of the dice and fate.
No customers came in; it was late and Jim Bob closed the diner while Thompson ate.

The beer was followed by another and another; Jim Bob said he was dying; it was ok; he was not crying.
He was sad, Thompson had been asking about the rib sauce; it was fantastic and he was not lying.

Jim Bob said he was closing the diner at the end of the week and would sell his recipe; he was close to tears.
He wanted three hundred dollars for it. It had been in the family for over sixty years.

Thompson said he would buy it and promised to return the next day with the money.
The next day he returned, bought the formula; Jim Bob gave him the mixing barrels and equipment too.

Jim Bob asked if Thompson would keep the name of the sauce the same.
Jim Bob had no family and the sauce was his only claim to fame.

Thompson's wife, Mary Jane thought it was another dream that would turn bad.
He said he would continue the two shifts a day work schedule; she was glad.

Thompson was not a gifted man, but he did finish the eighth grade.
He worked hard, never lost a job; he dared to dream, one good dream and he had it made.

Most people know the story about coke, the guy told him to bottle it.
Thompson designed the labels; Jim Bob's Rib and Barbeque Sauce was a hit.

To the boys at the pool hall, at the church fellowship meeting, he became a sage.
California was the new market and southern sauces were the rage.

Thompson started buying land and bought a number of small farms.
He was careful with a dollar, watched investments with the eye of a born horse trader; did not believe in charms.

The Jim Bob sauce continued year after year and Thompson finally sold out to Mr. Big.
Poor old Jim Bob sold for three hundred, died; Thompson sold for nine million and danced a jig.

Thompson Jr. knew, even hoped his dad would not make it to his sixty-fifth birthday party.
The years past swiftly and the party was two years away and Thompson Jr. was acting less than smarty.

Peggy Sue was still talking big party with her mother on the line, and in her mind thinking pine box all the time.
She was beginning to worry; dad was drinking less beer and every time she saw him, he looked fine.

Robert Lee was still the sheriff and the new doctor tells them to keep trying
His wife and he were planning on the big party and prayed dad would not be dying.

Thompson on his sixty-fifth birthday "Big Party" gave a little speech. Each and every one of his family was there. Mary Jane with all her family was very happy, let Thom preach

The family went to shower and change for dinner; it was a black tie affair.
Robert Lee and his dad, Thompson stayed outside to smoke a cigar in the fresh air.

Robert Lee was worried about his dad who was laughing so loud; afraid he would have a stroke.
His dad settled down and Robert Lee said, "Let me in on the funny joke".

Robert Lee you know your brother and sister were making bets that I would not be here this day.
I will tell you the joke, but please don't ever give it away.

Last year an attorney called; he asked me to visit his office, that was forty miles south, at no fee.
I was adopted and my real father had died at the age of ninety-two; he left eighty thousand dollars to me.

My Father had left a note saying his life had ended with my birth.
The note said, "Son, your Mother died in childbirth. I made arrangements with a good family and I am sorry for what it is worth".

The attorney said the truth should never be told and I agreed.

I laughed and cried with dad; we agreed to not tell the others, there was no need.

February 11, 1999

THE TEACHERS IN EDUCATION

(as I saw it)

Grand Mother was a School Teacher and I loved her
Those that are dedicated are great; some should not bother

On the average, I would give them the benefit of the doubt, and a grade of "B-"
The best of them, more than people think, make up for the worst, they get the title Finest

The Finest are not that hard to find, they are first-off intelligent, interested and kind
They are not usually the best dressers or the best groomed, but they have a sharp mind

Almost all are prim and proper, leaders who set good examples to the students, as well
The finest are not seeking rewards or notoriety in this life, as far as I can tell

They take joy in the little progress, shown by the slow students
And the knowledge that they could well be shaping some future Presidents

The thumper philosophy acknowledged, some teachers are very plainly bad

It would not be American, if all were the finest, to mention the others would be sad

The worst of the lot may be some of the world's top intellectuals, with no frills
Some of the greatest teachers are among the vast majority, in God-given skills

The Catholic Grammar School I attended, was a great school, all the teachers were dedicated nuns
They were interested and they showed it, not a worry about their rewards, they cared and still had fun

My grades were good; I was one of the top students in the class
High School was a different story; in my classes it was my goal to simply pass

Unfortunately, I started on the wrong foot; it was easy to blame the teacher
My first year of algebra, my grade was a "B+"; I created a little fuss, I was no preacher

The teacher was also the coach who had cut me off the baseball team
I was not a very good baseball player, not the worst but near the bottom of the stream

I asked the coach what the difference was between an "A-" and a "B+"
I will never forget his answer, "There is no difference, Piatt. I just gave you a B+"

The truth is, I was accustomed to receive top marks in all my math courses
My final words to the coach became my motto in high school, "O.K. coach, if you don't care, I don't care"

There were a few bad teachers in my seventeen years of going to school
Some of them were very, very good, a few bad, and one fool

The fool was the professor who taught law at Arizona State University
He was a CPA and a lawyer who felt he could walk on water, a pity

The test scores he posted, there were two; I was near the top, second or third, on the first test
The final, I had a grade of 92%. Number one in a class of thirty-five, it was the highest

The final grade he gave me was a "C"; I had an A grade average in my major
When asked, he said, "I had an 89% average, I had two class cuts and three times late

My average was one of the highest in the class, but he said I earned only a "B"
He docked me a grade for the cuts and late, like coach, an ego problem, my grade stood at "C"

You would think that the point could be argued, but I didn't care
The man was ignorant, pompous and unable to be fair

He saw my ability, thought I did not care, which was in part true
I was an honor student in college, an elected member of the Blue Key National Honor Fraternity, too

A grade is important, but many teachers play God with the power, they detest God-given knowledge of genius
The grace you earn is not yours by right, power can lower it to fit their ego, it is finished

A high school friend, a college fraternity brother, graduated from University of Arizona Law School
He would have had the highest grade point average ever, except one professor gave him a grade of "C"

My friend was a student, earned an "A"; the professor decided he did not deserve the number one spot
He showed his power by the grade he gave, he would decide who was and was not

In my freshman year of high school, there was an exceptional teacher
She taught Latin and English; I was fortunate to have her in both classes, she was one neat creature

She was special, caring and sharing, a leader and a listener, tough
I was happy when she gave me a "C" in both classes, I learned, the classes were rough

In first grade my teacher was great, a big, tall, and imposing woman who loved her job
You would think she would scare first graders; she made them feel important, needed, she was not a snob

There was a first grade candy sale; she gave me the job of making change, because I was so good with numbers
The compliment was never forgotten, and I remember it this day, positive ways were hers

My second and third years of high school, grade "B", the English teachers were young, pretty and caring
They related to each individual and to the class, they were special, both deserve the brass ring

The Catholic nuns were all dedicated, capable, caring, intelligent teachers
The Mother Superior, who taught seventh and eighth grades, the most understanding, and the finest award is hers

My high school years were four years of great fun and, like my grammar school days, rewarding
There were so many things I liked to do, from crawdad fishing to grand opera, happy days all worth recording

There were things that I would change, Mother Superior told Curly Rouse, the High School Principal
That she was sending a special student, an intellect and a leader to him from her 1948 class, I was despicable

My father told me the story, many years after he had heard it from his friend, Mr. Rouse; it made me sad
Mr. Rouse had told my father that, it was the first time, Mother Superior had been wrong; it made father feel bad

The second year Algebra class was very small, I was out of place with an attitude, I didn't care
The teacher, an attractive, intelligent lady, who cared and was ever so fair

She gave us a tough test, they all were, and she was happy to point out that I was the only one with the correct solution
The students were in the top of the class, except for me, I put the answer on the board; I appreciated the ego enhancing recognition

It seems to me that I really appreciated a little recognition and a pat on the back
The good teachers had a way of making everyone in the class feel special from time to time, a known fact

An excellent teacher and a nice person, pretty and intelligent was in my bookkeeping class, I had a crush
She wrote in my yearbook that she did not know anyone who goofed off in high as much as I did, it was true, but I did not blush

My final grade was "B", along with a compliment that I showed that I could do the work
She recognized and acknowledged my ability, but didn't like my acting the part of the jerk

The Track Coach was a special man; the Rinky Dink Coach was a special man, too
There was not one event in track that I could compete in; I was sad, but it was true

I was hooked on sports at a very early age; I truly loved competition, games and chess, too
Vade, Herb and I attended baseball, football, basketball, track, and I played golf, too

We went to out of town events in Phoenix, Tucson and Flagstaff, when we could
One runner, it was a thrill to watch, won state championships in the 100, 220, 440 and the hurdles, the decathlon, he should

The fourth year English teacher was a great teacher, recognized that I had a bad attitude and did not care
He had a sense of humor, smiled and laughed freely, wrote in my year book "There is a real world out there"

I always knew that there was a real world out there, but if people don't care, I don't care
Games, I like to play, I do not like to waste my time with people who cheat, or those who are not fair

It is not my intention to waste my life, only write my name in the sand
I hear more music than those who play in a one-man band

The real world is for those who care, are fair and create
They are teachers, firemen, postmen, shoeshine boys and Heads of State

They are members of a two hundred piece band; they each contribute to the music they play
Each member adds to the sound, if you listen you can hear the sounds of many yesterdays, today

The music they play is the building block of knowledge forever more
They all read music, contribute, care, share, are fair and know the score

September 8, 1998

THEY WERE A TEAM

We were students in a small Catholic Elementary School
The total enrollment was 222; we wanted to play Fourth Ave. Grammar School, cool

That year, 1946, they had an enrollment of twelve hundred and thirty four
We planned and schemed to beat them once more; this time more important than the win before

The team had Billy Lackie, Bobbie Stone, Hank Redondo, and the rest, all good players
Before the season was over, we were all good prayers

Hank and Ike were classmates, grade four through eight
We attended Yuma Union High and both graduated; it was fate

Arizona State University was the next stop in life's eternity
Vade Long and Mike Bierly, Hank and Ike all joined the same fraternity

Mike was from Columbus, Ohio and Yuma was home for the other three
We played poker, threw dice, partied day and night, and thought ourselves free

We lived in two apartments, behind the landlord's house; they were new and nice
Thankfully, Hank and I lived in the clean one, Vade and Mike cleaned theirs, but once or twice

The apartments were divided by a walkway and we never locked the door
We all agreed that two refrigerators were not needed so kept a keg in one evermore

We lived the good life as we did in high school, the best four years
We attended classes most of the time, did homework some times, and drank beer, Cheers!

Our first year of college was a terrible joke on us, each one
None of us made our grades, we were all capable, just plain dumb

Vade was drafted and Ike volunteered so Vade would not fight the war alone
We survived sixteen weeks of infantry training and took eight weeks of advance training

We were elite infantry soldiers; we were trained killers
We had changed little; we were drill sergeants, but not army pillars

We ended up in Germany as part of the U. S. Army Occupational Force
Mike was drafted shortly thereafter, lost his deferment and was drafted, of course

While we were defending our country, we all agreed, we all know war is hell
Hank moved to San Diego; he left school and went to work as well

After the battles, Vade, Mike and Ike laid aside their sharp blades
Battle-hardened veterans; they took school serious and made excellent grades

After graduation, Ike moved to San Diego and became Hank's roommate for the second time
In time there were three Redondo brothers and Ike; we all worked and got along just fine

Hank and Ike have been life-long friends and are close to this day
We see each other at reunions, exchange frequent calls and we did it the easy way

Back to the basketball championship of 1946; we were on a spin
I was the team captain and coach; we needed one last win

We had won all of our games to date; we had beat Fourth Avenue the first game
Defeated Jim Headington and his Crane School Team; it was no shame

We traveled to Somerton, near the old Mexico border
We clearly won the game and were ahead all the way, but their coach said the scoreboard was out of order

The little kid coach undaunted said that no matter what their coach said, "We Won!"
I gave him a thumbs up, and told him that winning had been fun.

The city championship game was at the Fourth Avenue School
We were well-trained and ready, our coach was no fool

We said our prayers and gave it our best effort, but we lost; some think it was fate
Our coach was to blame — he benched himself in the second half, but too little too late

They had forty or more players on their team
We had but nine players with a dream

August 6, 1998

THE RUNNER

The runner is a special athlete. The short distance runners require the God-given talent of speed. Without the gift a man can never be swift in the dashes. A long distance runner needs the gift too, but training and desire are required ingredients to make a champion. You cannot make a runner without the gift. You can be educated without being gifted. The most intelligent students are not recognized as such. They must fit the mold and do as they are told. They are held back. We have undoubtedly lost the benefit of genius in many fields, because it was not recognized. Einstein survived in spite of non-recognition of genius.

If you have a 100-yard dash man who runs the race in 9.3 seconds, you put him in uniform, encourage him to run and enjoy watching him run. He has to run in the lanes, cannot jump the gun and follows the basic rules. He can run as fast as he can.

In horseracing, they sometimes make the horses carry a required weight. We don't require the fast runner to carry a weight. Teachers grade gifted students down if they feel they are not doing their best. It is too easy for them, is an excuse, to require them to do more. In effect, they are required to carry a weight.

Runners don't always run their fastest possible race. They sometimes coast to a win when the next runner is far behind. They may settle for a third in a qualifying run, where the top three qualify.

A student who has studied Latin and Greek for eight years should not be required to take a language in high school or college. He should be tested by a standard test out of the classroom by an independent testing service. He should be given credit for the courses he is qualified for through testing. Many dollars can be saved by not requiring qualified students from taking a class in a subject he has mastered. There are cases where students are more knowledgeable than their teachers. Life could pass a little slower and time should be treasured, not wasted.

Professors with a PhD in Law and a CPA certificate should have more important things to do than keep track of students who are tardy three times in a semester.

MEXICALI, MEXICO – THE BULLFIGHT

Yuma, Arizona is only fifty miles from Calexico, California. Calexico is across the border from Mexicali, a short walk through the border inspection stations on both sides. The Mexican police, as you enter Mexico, wave you through with a serious expression that seems to say, "Don't give us any trouble." The United States border patrol asks you where you were born and what you are bringing back from Mexico. Don't be smart with them — they take their jobs seriously. They are thoroughly trained and pick up on the smallest things. They detect accents and nervous behavior where the keenest observer would not notice a thing.

The place to take your date for dinner or a date of special merit was Mexicali. We were juniors and seniors in Yuma High School in 1951 and 1952 and we made the trip five or six times a year. We would have a pleasant dinner in a first class nightclub for about five dollars each. Cocktails were sixty cents and they served anyone who could pay for the drinks. We sometimes went to a Chinese restaurant there with our parents. Alley Nineteen was the restaurant and the Chinese food was very good. Dinner there was less than three dollars and a quart of Mexicali beer was less than a dollar.

I was told as a youngster to respect the police. They had a tough job and were always right even when they were wrong. Treat them with respect and never challenge one doing his duty as an officer. You can challenge them in court at a later time if they are wrong but go through the channels. A "Yes sir" can save you a lot of hurt. A good friend of mine, on a boys' only trip, answered the border patrol officer as we left Mexico question with a funny one liner. My buddy did not mean to be disrespectful, but he was out of line. The border patrol officer asked him if he was bringing anything back from Mexico. He replied, "God, I hope not."

The officer was cool, said, "You're one of those guys; pull the car over there." The officer took the car apart, seats out, emptied the trunk, took the hubcaps off; checked the car end to end. The officer explained that they took their jobs seriously. We learned a little that day.

Two couples from Yuma decided to go to the San Diego Mountains to play in the snow one Saturday in December 1952. It never snows in Yuma, hardly once in fifty years. We take the same road as through Calexico, so on our way back we had dinner in Mexicali. When we stopped to clear the border after dinner, the border patrol officer asked me to open the trunk. They did this to one out of every three or four cars. I smiled, shook my head, and tried to keep a straight face. I told the officer, "You will not believe this sir." I opened the trunk and rapidly told him that I had promised my girlfriend's little brother that I would bring him some snow. The trunk was full of snow.

The border patrolman said, "How do I know what is under the snow?"

I said, "You don't sir, but I can dig it out in a minute."

The officer rolled a snowball, called a fellow officer and said, "Look at this!" They had a good laugh. The officer said, "Be on your way." He threw the snowball at his friend. They are under a lot of pressure and have a difficult job to do. Be nice, a yes sir or a no sir does not hurt, and they treat you with the same respect.

This day we were going to the Mexicali bullring to see a bullfight. Contiflas was famous as an entertainer in Mexico and this day he was fighting a bull. I had never seen a bullfight and this was my first. Contiflas was a Mexican movie star who was best known for his role in Around the World in 80 Days. He actually could fight bulls, but what we saw that day was a charade.

They had three fights before Contiflas fight. The pomp and ceremony is exciting and the parade of bull fighters and picadors is impressive. The matador is dressed in tights and very colorful. The pants are form-fitting and shiny with what looks to be mother-of-pearl flakes. The matador is said to stuff paper and other material in his crotch to appear bigger than life. They look like an oversized ballet dancer.

The first three bulls were impressive and almost noble beasts and were very formidable when let into the ring. They pawed the ground, snorted, their heads back and moved with grace and were swift. The assistant bullfighters taunted the bull for the first four or five passes. They did not venture far from their hole in the wall, as when the bull threatened them, they went behind the wall. It was their job to test the bull so that the matador could watch the moves of the bull. Each bull hooked a different way, raised or lowered its head a different way, the bullfighter needed all the information he could get.

The picadors plunged a lance into the shoulder muscles of the bull so the bull could not hook the matador so easily. The crowd booed the picadors as the bull attacked the picador's horse. The horse is covered on the side by a heavy blanket to keep the bull from tearing the horse's side open. It is a bloody sight not pleasant to watch. Just like the Roman Coliseum, the crowd reacts to the sight of blood. They cheer each pass by the matador and roar when the bull brushes by the fighter. They are excited by the closeness of the bull's horns. They cheer when the bull knocks the bull fighter down, but hold their breaths, if he appears hurt.

The kill is the most crucial part of the fight. The matador uses a sword to plunge through the bull's back and into the heart. He does this by going over the horns and if it is a good kill the sword severs the backbone and is thrust through the heart. There are a few seconds that the bull can seriously hurt or kill the matador. We saw the bull knock down one matador that day, but there were no serious injuries.

One fight, the bull struggled around the ring for a few minutes that seemed like an hour. The sword had been rammed to the hilt, but the bull refused to die. They finally were able to take a dagger and penetrate the spinal column at the base of the skull. The bull dropped like a sack of potatoes. The reward for a good fight, and especially a good kill, is an ear. Two ears, if the fight was more than good and a tail was thrown in for a great fight. No one was to receive the tail that day.

The crowd drinks and a good portion of the crowd is under the influence. Leather wine bags "Botas", are carried by many and they squirt a stream of red wine into the mouth, sometimes down the front and stains the shirt. The drinkers are probably ashamed to watch the bloody fight without courage from a bottle. Some are just tourists like us, looking for something to do. Many of the ladies do not watch the kill and only watch a small part of the fight.

Enter the great killer of bulls, Contiflas. He parades out to the center of the bullring and his pants fall down; he trips and falls on his face. The Mexican Charlie Chaplin is putting on a show. His act continued as he pulled up his pants. He is very talented and somewhat funny. The bullfighting is not a funny event and his antics were out of place, especially at the end of his act.

The announcer called for the bull and into the arena charged a young bull, about two-thirds the size of the previous bulls. The bull needed another year to grow into a fighting bull. Contiflas made a few passes with the bull. The bull easily tired and Contiflas grabbed the bull by the tail and threw the bull down. He laid on the bull and pulled out a comic book and read a few pages. The whole fight seemed to be a joke, but for one thing. It was hard to believe, but in the end, he took a sword and acted like he was going to kill the baby bull. He followed the sword over the horns and plunged the sword to the hilt in the bull.

He missed the spine; he missed the heart, but succeeded in puncturing a lung. The bull died a slow death. The fighter had the idea that it would be funny, if he pulled the sword out six or seven inches and made a big show of plunging it in again. The crowd hissed, some laughed, but we were disgusted. Our experience was on the low end of the entertainment scale and not the least bit funny.

I don't know why, but I did go again while on a trip to Spain, years later. I was curious and thought that the fights I saw were in some way flawed. The fights in Spain were much better, but it still is a bloody and cruel sport. I have no desire to see another.

February 2, 1999

We wander through life, see the sights, but seldom take the time to record the trip.

SCOTTSDALE, ARIZONA COCK FIGHTS

Watch out for that rooster, he has a knife. The rooster fights for his life. We were in college, at Arizona State University in Tempe. It was Saturday and we were looking for something to do. The story about a cock fight in Scottsdale, four or five miles north of Tempe, was being told around campus. The four of us thought it would be a way to pass a few hours and maybe learn something. Not one of us had seen a cock fight, did they wear gloves?

We were aware that it was against the law in Arizona to have cockfights and also against the law to be an observer at a cock fight. We broke a few laws in those days as the police thought the college kids were special and gave us every break possible. We pushed our luck a little in 1954.

You would think that a fight that was against the law would be held in a barn or a warehouse in the shady area of town. We were surprised that everyone in the greater Phoenix area knew about the cock fights. You might think that the police were also aware. We followed the directions and were amazed to see a miniature coliseum, designed like the coliseum in Rome, but in a much better state of repair. The building was single wall construction and built out of plywood, it would not stand long. The inside had seating around a circular fighting ring. The place was almost full and we managed to find a seat in the back. All of the seats had an excellent view of the fighting arena.

The girls were outwardly very nonchalant and all grown up, but they had never seen a cock fight. They would soon turn a little yellow and then white as the night progressed. The four of us were amazed at the swift pace of the night. It was as if everyone had an uncontrollable desire to give away all their money. The betting was at a frantic pace and the feathers flew.

A fight featured a rather pretty gold and red rooster pitted against a yellow and black rooster. Two lines were drawn in the dirt center of the arena. They were about three feet apart. The roosters were tended by a handler who was like a cut man for a heavyweight title fight. They could almost bring a rooster back from the dead. They actually gave the roosters mouth-to-mouth resuscitation, at times, if necessary. They are fanatics and don't like to lose.

The stakes are in the hundreds and maybe in the thousands. The betting starts at five dollars for the students and other poor folks. The arena is run by a pit boss, who sets the preliminary odds and changes the odds as the fight progresses. We were soon to find out what a cockfight was. The pit boss was a short slight man of Mexican descent and he must have a PhD in odds-making and the eye of an eagle. He moves around the ring making bets while the fight is going on. He stands on a box in the ring at the start of the fight when he sets the preliminary odds.

The pit boss may make fifty or sixty bets during the one to two minutes each fight takes. The odds are changed after each flare up of the fighters, as he sees, or thinks he sees, something that indicates the style or the inflicted damage of the roosters has changed. Some betters offer a bet on odds they like and the bet is either accepted or declined with a nod or head shake. The pre-fight odds were eight to five on the gold rooster. The roosters are fitted with a circular spur on each leg. The spur is a one-half inch razor sharp knife. The roosters flair or jump straight up, flap their wings; kick their legs and try to cut their opponent.

The handlers use two hands to hold the birds before the first flare up. The fighters are introduced by rubbing their heads together. They are each placed behind the line facing one another. Released, the roosters jump up, lean back and start kicking. It is fast and only the trained eye can detect the first signs of skill or injury to the fighting cocks. The odds are changed to six to five on the gold rooster. They hit the ground and instantly jump again, kicking and spurring and the knives flash. The odds change to six to five in favor of the black rooster. The odds change five to six more times in the next minute.

It is apparent that the gold rooster is hurt, his head is bloody and the fighters seem to have

forgotten where the other bird was. The trainers pick up their fighters for another face off. They blow down their throats, one sucks the blood out of his fighters throat and spits it out at ringside. The gold fighter can lift his head up only slightly and appears to be unable to see. The birds are ready for the final face off. They are put on the line facing each other and released. The gold rooster stands square to the line, cannot see and does not flare. The yellow and black rooster backed off the line.

He has had enough and has the fight won, but quick as a flash; his owner kicks him in the head and kills him. The yellow and black rooster was disqualified and lost the fight when he backed off the line. The crowd was heated as those who bet on the gold rooster collected their bets. The pit boss walked around the ring and collected twenty bets and paid off thirty bets. He had made over fifty bets at odds different for each bet and never wrote one down. The five fights we watched, he never made a mistake. A remarkable talent wasted on what turned out to be my one and only visit to a cockfight.

I am sure our dates were sick and would never return to a cockfight again. The fights last only a minute or two each, but it does not take a college student more than one fight to know the fights should be against the law. Arizona has grown up a lot in the last fifty years, but they probably have a fair number of people who like to raise and fight chickens.

DATELAND 1956

On July 6, 1956, I was driving on Highway 80 between Phoenix, Arizona and Yuma, Arizona. It was a hot day. I passed through Gila Bend, when it was 106 degrees in the shade. The map showed it was fifty miles from Gila Bend to Dateland.

Dateland had two service stations and both had restaurants. One station and one restaurant had closed years before. Dateland was a favorite stopping place for us, who knew the road. It was 70 miles to Yuma from Dateland.

The service station in Dateland did not have a sign in the window. A nicely dressed black man stepped out of a clean, but older station wagon. He had the look of a college professor, with three children, ages 6, 8, and 10, and a well dressed wife. He was from Alabama. He asked to see the manager. The manager introduced herself and said, "It is a typical hot day. What can I do for you?"

The black man asked, "Could I bring my family in for a cool drink?"

"Would this table be ok? Please bring your family in. It is terribly hot outside."

August 3, 2006, at 4:24 in the afternoon, he told me that He had a message for me. My Bible was open. He instructed me to add 11 to the page you are reading (11 + 423 = 434). I turned to that page 434, and it contained, "The last years and death of Judith".

I was married twice. Twenty-one years to my first wife and seventeen years to the second. I had many times told Him, that I did not like living alone.

God made man and the desire to multiply is strong. I don't like living alone, but have nothing to offer. Parkinson's robs me of my energy, speech, writing ability, hopes, and desires fade away.

Dressing is a job. I sit on the floor to put my pants on. I try to write, but struggle. I am getting a little more energy — slowly. The "cancer killing seeds" have been implanted for two years next month. The radioactive Iodine seeds kill good cells and bad. They are left in for life. What strength I had left, they took.

God has seen me through some tough times. Miracle and another miracle, God has worked to save me. I forget to thank Him for emergency treatment, accidents that should have killed me many new medical techniques, medicines, etc., that have saved me.

MATERIALITY

Life goes on into infinity
But it is all too short for you and me

We, my friends, are but a second in the life of man
So why do we worry, sweat and toil to draw a picture in the sand

You must work long and hard to acquire your material wants
But if you work too long and too hard, it may be too late to enjoy one little pleasurable jaunt
Study hard, so what! —

I WAS A CHRISTIAN

Endowed with a play disposition
It was July 6, 1956, one hundred years after the Civil War
The war to abolish slavery
Over 500,000 men fell to free the Blacks
Brother fought brother
The "no colored trade solicited" stayed
In Yuma, Arizona, the city plunge in which no blacks played
The Yuma Movie Theatre admitted Blacks
They sat in the balcony with the Indians
The Fourth Avenue Grammar School admitted Blacks
They went in the side door to the basement
Give credit to the Immaculate Conception Catholic School
They encouraged Blacks; a great school, but no pool
Written in 1957, in my Advanced Accounting textbook inside the cover

Many of my old poems were saved. I was a poet long before saving my work.

OUR SHORT LONGEVITY

So we see
What is to be

But still we try
Until we die

Enjoy yourself; it is later than you think
In the eyes of time, birth to death is but a wink

COLLEGE

Rain, the day is quiet, music is soft, Sunday
Tomorrow we start fresh again, blue Monday

Years, five, have past since we started this task
Many a cheery time, football games, balls, have past

You and I, my soul, have been so free and carefree
Cold, cloudy, quiet Sundays bring a question to you and me
What does the future show us to be

We work for what we see not
For something we haven't got

If and when, we find what we are looking for, at last
Will we, soul and I, find satisfaction in these years past

Rain, the day is quiet, music is soft, Sunday
Tomorrow, fulfillment we may find, someday

November 16, 1998

OLD DOCTOR JOE

Dr. Joe was never too busy or important to return a call
He made house calls day or night, in winter, spring, summer or fall

Most Doctors gave up house calls; fees were increased, by stacking appointments in their office suite
A family doctor was good old Joe, dependable, very knowledgeable, capable and sweet

Proud of his work and his ability to spot trouble
An internal medicine diagnostic specialist, he loved to burst trouble's bubble

He studied medicine at the University in Texas, an excellent school
He was a good family man, a great internist; he was no one's fool

Instrumental in starting the Goleta Valley Hospital, he was misled by a foe
Old Dr. Joe entrenched and prepared for an all out war, he was ready to fight toe to toe

It took a lot of swearing, sweating and fretting to avert a total loss
There were a lot of friends, who had invested, who would have gone down too; but Joe was the boss

He won the war, but he was deeply hurt by the attempt to bankrupt the hospital and it's supporters too
Dr. Joe was a leader, who did what he had to do

Old Dr. Joe was a fighter, but his main foe was illness
A family Doctor, true to his oath, made house calls, but not under duress

Was he a Doctor or a Friend? He was both to his patients and friends
Medicine was his first passion, but he loved to play until the end

The other passions were family, the piano, song and he also liked a drink or two
At party time, it was not unexpected for Dr. Joe to play all night through

He had a friend across the street, who had a grand piano, too
Dr. Joe stopped by, played the piano in a grand style and had a drink or two

For the great conversation, piano, and medical advice, he was given a key
Dr. Joe visited many times over the years; any excuse would do —
Like a dog barked or he was bitten at home by a flea

Old Dr. Joe liked to say Hello and most always had a joke to tell
But the first and lasting passion was to make the sick well

He was a little city family Doctor, a big-hearted Doctor from Texas who cared
We, who remember, are forever grateful for the gifts he so gracefully shared

CRUSCKOVE'S VISIT (1961 OR 1962)

During his brief span of years, there are many times when a man must wonder.
When freedom, liberty, family, or friends are threatened, should man be a pacifist and sit calmly by or
Should he adorn himself with a warriors cloak, pick up a stick and face the threatening thunder?

Is it a wise, prudent man who always remains in the middle of the street?
True, a man in this position may at all time proceed or retreat.

A pacifist may be friend or foe.
You probably will never know.

A man always neutral seldom has a worthwhile friend.
Much better a friend who acts, who speaks his mind,
And who makes commitments upon which friendship truly must depend.

Pacifism and neutrality are useless friends when one's liberty, country and family are menaced by a foe.
When in need, friends speak up, align with you, side by side, they pledge you their support and then you know.

He had proved to be your friend
For a time your wondering may end.

These are grave times. Man is faced with a distant visitor, a malignant monster.
The monster's hand hovers menacingly, threatening — no, promising to unleash a grotesque,
Meandering friend more devastating than all, contained in the bottomless pits of Lucifer.

After much wondering, you stand in warrior's cloak, willing to face and fight this ever spreading malignancy alone.
During times of lesser crisis, your friends quarreled with you, laughed at you, at times even chastised you,
But today — today, they joined by your side and united man and friends drove the thundering malignancy home.

There are many times when a man must wonder.
If enough friends unite they can quiet the fear of, and drown the thunder.

MY LIFE WITH SARAH, MY 2nd WIFE

The date was May 8, 1984. Sarah and I had dinner, danced, and drank four brandies. We fit, shared many of the same interests and I was in love. I had met her nineteen years before.

Clyde was born February 11, 1934 and was 69 years old. Sarah was born June 14, 1940 and was 63 years old. They lived in Camino Melena, Rancho Del Ciervo Estates in 1967 as neighbors. Clyde bought his home there and Sarah's home was two doors up the street.

Today the houses sell for over one million dollars. Clyde lived there until April 1982, 15 years. His first wife, Roberta sold the home in 1984-85, for $400,000.

Clyde lived in an apartment in Santa Barbara, from 1982 until August 1985, when he moved in with Sarah. Sarah rented out two bedrooms to two separate golfers, after her husband died about 1983. She rented out the maid's quarters to a young lady. Sarah's home was over 3,000 square feet and was sold for $250,000 in 1989. Today's fair market value is over $800,000.

Clyde and Sarah bought a home in Lake Wildwood, California, in a gated community, country club and golf course. The association also owned one of the largest private lakes in California. The home was on Echo Blue Drive, Penn Valley, California. We bought the home jointly.

Sarah's Mother, Mrs. Masterson, paid $300,000 towards the Buckeye Court home, purchased in April 1991, for $350,000. Sarah added a T.V. room and a hidden room. The addition cost $50,000+.

We bought a $3,000 T.V. and added $15,000 in new heating systems and stoves. The home was purchased new. It was almost 4,000 square feet. This home has a market value today of over a million dollars. We lived there over five years.

Sarah had an on and off way with her Mother, Mrs. Masterson. We left Santa Barbara because of her Mother. We left Lake Wildwood because of Mrs. Masterson. Sarah was determined to get away. We planned a trip and ended up on an extended vacation, 3 years in Alabama, 3 years in Arizona. We were expecting Mrs. Masterson to die. It was rumored, she drank a fifth of Vodka a day and inhaled prescribed drugs, uppers and downers.

I believed that Sarah would be happy and the war with her Mother would be over. I knew we would have some good years and enjoy ourselves.

LOVE...

It may happen quickly
Like "love at first sight"
Or slowly, through sharing,
But either way's right.
For what really matters
Is that you've found love
And with it, more joy
Than you've ever dreamed of!
We have something very special ~
I'm so glad you came into my life!
Happy Easter
Yours and only Yours
I Love You
Sarah
XXXXXX

July 5, 1985
My Darling Ike
… BUT I'LL GIVE YOU
'TIL AROUND THE
YEAR 2999…
Yours and Only Yours
I Love You
Sarah
XXXOXX
See you and John tonight.

7/11/85
It's just Me, wanting you to know you are with me in
my heart, my dreams, my thoughts, my soul,
my Fantasies, and on my mind every minute
of the day and night.
I love you,
Yours and Only Yours — Sarah
XXXXXXOXX

July 22, 1985
When I am working, you are with me
When I am playing, you are with me
When I am alone, you are with me
Even though we may be apart
You are always with me

Sometimes it still amazes me — how I get so anxious and thrilled and thoughtful about you;

I guess maybe it's because I just keep falling wonderfully in love with you…over and over again.

With All My Love
Yours and Only Yours
Sarah

July 29, 1985
How can I put it delicately?
My Darling Ike
Falling in love with you
was the best idea I ever had!
Thank You Sweetheart
Yours and Only Yours
Sarah
XXXXOXXOXX
See you tonight if you feel like it.July 31, 1985

You can't have everything Sweetheart
I love you
XXOXXXO
From
Yours and Only Yours
Me

Darling Ike,

I'm not sure when I first fell in love with you… I guess it could have been as early as that first time we held each other, or the first time I realized that you kind of liked me, too…I'm not sure, I just remember thinking of you more and more and getting less and less done in the process! I remember wanting you to stay so badly ~ and being so thrilled at the thought. I remember praying that it was you whenever the phone would ring, but at the same time hoping it wasn't, because I didn't know how in the world I was going to sound romantic and impressive when what I felt was anxious and tongue-tied…

I love You, My Darling
See you this P.M.
Yours and Only Yours
Sarah
XXXXOXXXX

August 5, 1985
To my Darling Ike,

THANK YOU FOR GIVING ME THE PLEASURE OF GIVING PLEASURE TO YOU!

To trust in your love for me and pray that it grows stronger every day

To watch our love grow together through the years
I promise to soothe your mind and body
To plan with you, dream with you
To do my best to show you how much I love you
For you have become my world, my heart, my life

The future is ours… always~ *Excerpt by Jacqueline Dumas*
This says it All.
I love You
from
Yours and Only Yours,
Sarah
XXXXOXX

August 14, 1985
I promise you my love…
without any limits
To accept the things
you believe in
and to always try
to understand you
To be near you
whenever you need my presence…

Good Morning Darling
Thank you for staying over last night.
If you would like, you can stay tonight.
Now don't tell me that you were not asked.
I love you more than words can say.
From Yours and Only Yours,
XXXOXXXXX S.
I Love Mr. Piatt

August 15, 1985

Good Morning My Darling Ike

As always I love you, but I love you more than I did yesterday.

And I know I will love you more tomorrow.

I am truly Yours and Only Yours.

Have a Good Day. I will talk to you later this A.M. Call me when you can.

I miss You and love You.

Sarah

XXXOXXXOX

September 30, 1985

Good Morning My Darling

It's a new day, and I love you more than ever. You are a sweetheart. Thank you for loving me and making me feel so wanted and loved. I hope that I can only show you how much you are loved and wanted. Have a wonderful day. I will miss you. Please call if you have time.

Yours and Only Yours

Forever-

Sarah

XXOXOXO

I'm So Glad You're My Husband
"A husband is a special friend
who cares and shares and loves."
I love you for being a wonderful man
with so much love to share…
I love you for being a special friend
who shows such warmth and care…
I love you for being my partner through life
as only you could be…
I love you for being everything
that means the most to me.

Happy Birthday
All My Love
Yours and only yours
Sarah
XXXX
2-11-94

Sarah was in Mobile, Alabama in April of 1992. She was caring for her Father, who was dying of brain cancer. Here is her letter to me:

"Hi Sweetheart,

Just a line or 2, to let you know, how much I miss you, and love you. Nothing too new around here; he is not any better or worse. It makes a big difference having help in the a.m. and p.m. The cost is $8.25 per hour and is not covered by Medicare or his Blue Cross. I don't know why? Hopeful his money will last, so that he can have the care. Also there is a four hour minimum, so it adds up to 8 hours per day. He is more and more forgetting things, but remembers when is showed or driven by.

Talked to the other Banker yesterday and was told about Jimmy's visit to the bank. The Banker did not like what was going on and put a hold on Daddy's check. He said my Dad was very confused that day and was asking to do some things he had never done before, in the years he had done business with the bank in Mobile. But Jimmy was very insistent on Daddy cashing in two Federal Notes. Also wanted to know how soon the money would be returned. Makes me wonder what the hell else he did or got away with, when he was here???

Well that's about it, all the depressing days. I do love you and miss you more than words can say, and hope and worry about you being alone. I promise, I will make it up to you.

Take care and just remember you are the most wonderful man in the world and that I love you.

Yours and only yours,

Sarah xxxxxo"

In April 1996, Sarah said, "We are leaving Lake Wildwood". I agreed, since there was no real choice on my part.

When we moved from Santa Barbara to Lake Wildwood, Sarah had asked. I told her, "I had to work and would commute. Lake Wildwood to Santa Barbara is 465 miles".

Sarah was to make the trip with me many times. I was invited by Martha Masterson, in fact, she "insisted", that I stay with her. Over the next seven and a half years, I was to spend over 1,000 nights with Martha.

Martha was a character out of "Charles Dickens". She led an exciting life. For example, she rode the "Concord" to Europe from New York to London, on one of the first flights. She returned on the QE 2, after a week on the Oriental Express.

Martha was the victim of a murder threat in Scottsdale, Arizona. She carried a large suitcase of fake money at the drop point while the FBI followed. The money was never picked up.

Martha was in a bad section of town late at night. The area was the nightspot for black drug dealers. Martha was a beautiful, trim, red headed lady, who did whatever she damn well pleased. The three raped her. One of the men told Martha, "Run for it, they plan on killing you." She ran. The three rapists were caught and sent to prison.

Martha had a live-in boyfriend, John, a Catholic Priest, for over twenty years. She built Catholic churches, during her 86 years of life. She built "donated money" to the University of California in Santa Barbara. When Martha died, the flag was lowered to half mast at UCSB in her honor.

Martha, Mrs. Samuel B. Masterson, was reported to be one of the richest women in the world.Mrs. Masterson's next escort was a Monsignor in Los Angeles, California. Martha taped their conversation for over five years. The tapes described sex items. Martha enjoyed parties, dancing and was often wasted. She liked dancing with Clyde. Martha did not support Sarah. She told Clyde that she was not leaving Sarah a dime.

Martha did not like our modest home in Lake Wildwood. It had a long curvy driveway and was steep. Martha said, "It was dangerous, especially in snow and ice. Martha bought Sarah a new home in Lake Wildwood. It cost $300,000 and $25,000 paid out of escrow by Sarah. Sarah put $75,000 in improvements. The total cost was $400,000. It was a beautiful home with a view of the lake and golf course. We lived there until 1996.

Parkinson's slowed me down, but I continued to play golf. My handicap went from fifteen to twenty one over ten years. The last game I played was in 1997 at Gulf Park, Louisiana. I was determined to break one hundred and I shot a ninety-six. I was ten years into the fight at that time.

I still enjoyed eating out, going to the movies, and sex — life was still good. We are active in Jewish studies at the Spring Street Temple; both directors of Mobile, Alabama Kennel Club and had six dogs. Sarah showed the dogs. We traveled back and forth to Santa Barbara and were living a full life.

These were the medications I was taking when we moved to Alabama: Sinemet 29/100, every three hours and at bedtime as needed; Sinemet CR 25/100 in the evening and at bedtime as needed; and Tasmar 100y every six hours.

We drove to Mobile, Alabama for a few days visit and stayed three years until the hurricanes frightened us away.

QUEEN SUGAR BABE

Born early one cool crisp morning on the queen sugar plantation
She was an afghan pup, born with, a knowledge of her high station

Three thousand acres of primeval forest a private hunting ground
Ghosts, ugly beasts of every size, just waiting to be found

A pond of great size loaded with exotic fish, big, little and tiny
Her world as seen only by her was oh, so marvelous and ever shiny

Her mistress could not see the forest and only noticed the trees
Her mind was set on a world championship, not the birds and the bees

It is true Sugar strutted, was ever proud, arrogant, and beautiful
She was loving, caring, sharing and very dutiful

But she had her visions and longed to be what she was, an afghan pup
Pampered, brushed, and properly groomed, she won the puppy cup

There were more important things to do, dragons and beasts wait
The forest dark, sinister and spooky, challenged her fate

The pond and its fishes of every color and size
The numbers dazzle her; her life is a giant surprise

She was prepared for a great show, every hair in place
She had to get outside, the grooming had been at a snail's pace

The friends big and little called her; they wanted to play
The fish in the pond demanded time to add their say

The fun began with a chase of the dragons, a chase of the dark Sinister spooks too
The pond called and beckoned, so what could she do, into the water she flew

The Sugar Babe on a warm summer day chased goblins, went fishing, splashed and played
That day she was a puppy still, but her mistress had other ideas and prayed

She prayed that the Sugar Babe would grow up and win the cup
The prayers were answered suddenly, one day Sugar grew up

The prime evil forest, the elegant pond, and beasts big and little are gone away
The elegant pond is now but a little puddle, in the back yard, where Sugar, as a smiling, happy and gifted puppy, used to play

But she laughs as she remembers, the big day she was prepared for the show
She pretended nervously that she had to go

She chased her friends, tiny, shiny, big and little
Swam in the pond, then wet and muddied, she finally piddled

Her face wore a mischievous grin
It was a puppy's last spin

My first published poem, published in 1998, POETRY GUIDE "A CELEBRATION OF POETS" in the Flagstaff, Arizona Kennel Club News May/June, 2001

THREE SIGHT HOUNDS

The greyhound was with us first; she is five
Then we saved an afghan pup, we hope to survive

The greyhound was a professional racer; she could fly
The afghan we acquired from a rescue group, I wonder why?

We are Directors of the Mobile Kennel Club, we don't know how
We want to participate; my wife wanted a show dog now

She bought a Borzoi pup, a Russian wolfhound to me
That is how we acquired the sight hounds, three

The afghan is a loving and beautiful pup
It hurts a little to see her growing up

The Borzoi looks like Icabod Crane
A pup, skinny and the size of a great dane

My wife and I have morning coffee on the patio, while they play
They provide us with smiles and laughter to start the day

The greyhound, Cindy, runs at a great pace
The pups, Moisha and Sugar make it a three-dog race

Cindy retires and the pups start their roughhouse tricks
They jump, push, shove, knock each other down, get in their licks

Our little old lady, the silky, thinks the fight is real
We and the pups know it is all for fun and no big deal

The silky cries murder, we laugh and the pups play
For all except the silky, it's a pleasant way to start the day

August 8, 1998

DOG DAYS AND THE MISSUS

Naughty, not nice, she is gloom
Mobile dog days of summer, in bloom

July the 16th and it has been sticky, stormy and hot
The Missus has been sassy, mean, screaming and fought

She is mad, mean and mad. It is sad
I turned into a stammering cad

It seems the dog days of summer are in all ways here,
The dog days are numbered and they walk with fear

The dogs and I are in the boat together
We all wish we were birds of a feather

We could all sing the Misses blues away
If that fails, we could all fly the coop; it would make her day

The dog days of summer are surely to blame
Tomorrow we pray will be better, but expect more of the same

Time flies and so goes the summer
The dog days are certainly a bummer

BOMB AGAIN THIS DAY

This day, as referred to in the Bible, means today.
Religious fanatics set off the bombs and innocent people pay.

They die by the tens and hundreds for no reasonable reason.
On the way home or to pray, just taking a walk, anytime or any season.

They were not targeted; they were just there by chance.
The killers celebrate their death, yell and dance,

Better they and all the planners dance at the end of a rope.
Killing innocent people cannot be fun, yet they laugh and joke.

There is not a way to justify the random slaughter; it must end.
To kill God's people without reason is devil's work; the good it offends.

The killers are few in number; the bad they do is loud like thunder.
They get all the headlines they seek; no glory or pride do they receive, why? I wonder.

The dead include old and young, many varied religions, children as well.
The sick of mind, fanatics, mass murders, have been with us since the first bell.

Take every precaution, hang them when caught, and do a lot of praying.
We can slow them and kill a few; God can stop them, pray and give up fair playing.

August 8, 1998

AMERICA & PIE

Sailors today do not have Mother printed on their tattoo
In days gone by, it was quite the in thing to do

They do not preach Mom-ism and apple pie anymore
It is not as popular to wave the American Flag, as before

No one seems to care about communism; did it die?
We seem to be obsesses with putting satellites in the sky

Progress is great; we are making life easier every day
Of course, the wife now has to work, so the children can play

It is no longer a big deal for a family to see a ball game
It is not worth a weekend to visit the zoo; its' too tame

We have our great movies, Rocky II, Shoot I'm and Big Boom
The special effects, blood and mess, crashes, are but gloom

There are a few good family pictures still made, but very few
We need to retreat to the library, for learning and adventure, too

Mother would roll over in her grave at $135.00 for tennis shoes
If she knew the cost of visiting Disney Land or Magic Mountain, she would have the blues

Today children have rights too; we don't want them deprived or not given their due
Saying no to the child's requests will hurt their ego; it will kill the rainbows they pursue

What are good Americans; loving and caring persons, choices?
It is time to carry a big stick and make certain the children hear your voices

Restrict their choices, help them think, direct them, listen to them, too
Wave the flag, make them eat apple pie; let them know you are the leader and they are the crew
August 10, 1998

BLUE BIRDS ARE BLUE

People tell you to look at the bright side of your fears.
It is nighttime; you feel blue and shed a few tears.

Don't be a crybaby; it will pass soon.
You put on a fake smile and grin at the new moon.

The smile takes away none of the pain.
It makes others feel better all the same.

It is really true, you give it all you have; you try
You don't tell your friends; deep down you still want to cry.

There are some who think it is attention and sympathy you seek.
They don't understand that you are blue; you have never been weak.

Nothing in life is good anymore and you want to hide.
This has been going on for years and does not subside.

You used to drink and have fun;
Now you drink and have none.

So you quit drinking and going to a party is not for you.
You don't go anywhere, grow up and quit being blue.

Your son marries, but still you feel no joy.
No joy do you have when your daughter has a baby boy.

The neurologist runs a few tests. He knows your trouble.
The brain has a joy center and yours needs a dopa double.

Carbidopa, Paxil, Tasmar, and Permax combined and I feel fine;
Not high or low, just fine. Your mind is clear all the time.

This effect may not last forever.
You don't want the blues back ever.

No one should take a mind altering chemical; used to be good advice.
Properly prescribed, it makes the sick well and the nasty people nice.

You again smile and laugh at the right time.
The smile is back; there are mountains to climb.

Your son and daughter were sad when you felt bad.
They are ever pleased and you are glad

FOUR SIGHT HOUNDS

It appeared to be a joke, she mentioned it time and again; I soon suspected it was not a play
The Misses told me about expecting a new family member; our memory is not as good as yesterday

It took a few months, of short statements, but I managed a clear view
She has been a friend for thirteen years, what will she do tomorrow, I don't have a clue

We needed a change; our home in Mobile, Alabama has been a very happy place
Southern people are especially nice; the forest is green, a beautiful city; no more L.A. rat race

The weather is hard to beat, a storm or two, lets you know who is the boss
July in Mobile is hot, if anyone tells you it is not, they had too much sauce

The Misses is a little up in years, to have morning sickness
Yesterday was the delivery date, I voted, but it did not count, I'm but a witness

The arrival was a cause for celebration, one hundred drums and a marching band
What it lacked in quality, it made up in volume; it was the only band at hand

There were oh's and ah's a plenty, you had to fine tune to separate the sound
Our little 13 year old Silky, gave her meanest roar, tried to frighten the hound

Our nine-month old afghan hound, Sugar Babe, was a very happy pup
She pranced, danced, smelled and tested, then showed the eight week old pup his magical world with a strut

The sugar plantation was born anew, three thousand acres, all forest and sugar cane
The big pond returned, the creatures big, little, small and tiny returned, I'm glad they came

They played the National Anthem, while we stood silently by
I don't believe it happened, but it was plain to see, the baby had a tear in her eye

They went for a romp in the forest; happy as could be, the sight hounds four
It would be tempting fate if I entered a plea, "No Ma's for favor", please no more

Coffee bright and early overlooking the plantation, form our patio
It was all smiles and lively chatter as the sight hounds put on a rodeo

We forgot last night's puppy cries for his family far away.
With love, attention and affection, his loss will fade and he will be happy to stay

Cindy, the greyhound, Moisha, the Russian Wolf-hound, the Afghan
Ismial and Sugar, the royal family
It is a beautiful morning; the hurricane has gone away; life smiles on us, whatever will be, will be
October 4, 1998

CALIFORNIA TO NEW ORLEANS

We stayed in a historical old home in the French Quarter of New Orleans. It had been a large home with a central courtyard, a fountain and gardens. They had converted it into six units, three with sitting rooms and in three of the units, kitchens for the long-term visitor.

Elizabeth, the owner of the units was a long term resident of New Orleans; she smoked. To say she smoked was like saying New Orleans was a night city. She often had two cigarettes going at the same time, but always a minimum of one. A chain smoker, who did not light one cigarette with another, but never put one out without first lighting another.

She told us a dozen or two stories about the old days in the French Quarter. We learned that the building used to be three stories. It was now two. The third story was converted into a distillery during Prohibition. They had an explosion and that was the end of the third story. In a close room, the smell of the cigarette is bad especially to a non smoker, her breath was a reminder that death is waiting around the corner.

Elizabeth told us where to go in and about New Orleans. She gave us a list of restaurants that she recommended we try and a list that she recommended we do not try. She listed costs and service for each. She was entertaining and we agreed that she had probably raised a little Cain in her younger days.

My parents used the term, raising Cain, when I was a kid in Arizona. The saying probably owes its roots to Joe Cain, who is a hero in Mobile, Alabama. They celebrate Joe Cain, every year, as a part of the Mardi Gras. She listed a few tourist spots and said to go if we had to. The food was good ant the prices ridiculous, but if you must impress your friends; go.

Joe Cain Day is also celebrated in Nevada City and this year Nevada City people along with the President attended the party in Mobile. We may see people all over the United States raising Cain in the next few years. Joe Cain was reburied in a place designated at Poet's Corner in the old Mobile Cemetery.

We had driven from Lake Wildwood, located in the Sierra Mountains, California. We had stopped at the Louisiana information center as we entered the state. I made reservations at the Las Maisonette Apartments and looked over the maps available. A debonair gentleman was standing by our car and I said hello. He was direct and asked where we were from. I told him Santa Barbara, California where I still maintained an office and my wife said Grass Valley. Grass Valley is the best-known town in the area, where Lake Wildwood is located. Nevada City is three miles north of Grass Valley and it is in the Sierras north of Sacramento.

He introduced himself and said his name was Norm Randolph. He said he was from the same area. He asked where in Grass Valley we lived. My wife explained that we had recently moved to Lake Wildwood. Norm said that was where they lived too. Ned was on his way to visit New Orleans and I asked him if he had a place to stay. They did not and I recommended Las Maisonette; I called and made a reservation for them.

We chatted for a few minutes and I asked them to join us for dinner in New Orleans. They arrived as we were making our reservations and I asked if he would like to go to any special restaurant for dinner. He said he was not familiar and would leave it up to me. I suggested the Commander's Palace and made reservations for eight o'clock that evening.

Norm and his wife turned out to be one of the most interesting couples we had ever met. His wife was from Montecito, a upper class section of Santa Barbara, California. She was a lady and we soon found out that Norm was a sophisticated prankster. He was a gentle person who was happy acting the class clown. He said he was dying during a lull in the dinner conversation and his wife said, "Norm, you always tell people you are dying, but you eat well, enjoy your drinks and keep smiling."

We heard the same story a few more times the next year. Norm had been the youngest passenger on the Hindenburg's last flight, before it crashed and burned. He said that it was a great way to travel; everything was done in style. He was thought to be the only living passenger of that Hindenburg flight.

The dinner was over and it was time to leave. The bill was given to Norm and he said he was buying dinner. We had not made previous arrangements and I tried to pay the bill. I suggested the flip of a coin to decide and Norm lost. All four of us had such a good evening that I suggested breakfast in the morning. They were leaving after breakfast and I made a reservation at Brennan's.

Brennan's breakfast starts with a Bloody Mary, Champaign or a Silver Fizz and is a special treat. The conversation picked up with Norm dying and we enjoyed the shared stories. Norm was amazed at the cost of two eggs. The breakfast tab was almost the same as dinner the night before. This time no coin flip as I was buying. We have not seen them for a few years, but assume that Norm is still dying.

You need a good stomach and a healthy appetite to really appreciate New Orleans. We had black beans and rice, red beans and rice, blackened fish and blackened steak. You are able to relish two dozen oysters on the half shell each. The cherry stone clams, like the oysters, you eat raw. We tried them both fried, baked with spinach and in a gumbo.

The gumbo is a story in itself. Your taste will tell you it is great, but you don't fret over what the cooks put in it. A timid person may not be able to appreciate it if you describe the varied ingredients. The southern beer is delicious and helps to wash down some of the special treats such as crayfish. In Arizona, as a kid we called them crawdads. The gourmet can eat fifty or sixty crayfish in a normal lunch or dinner meal.

New Orleans is supplied with fresh seafood from Louisiana, Mississippi, and Alabama. The Gulf of Mexico is a fantastic provider and the fishermen keep the restaurants well supplied. The local people simply expect great seafood and they get it.

Bourbon Street is as it has been for many years, a tourist spot and a mad house of fun. They have a few murders each year, but seem to leave the good guys alone. The dope dealers shoot each other and do their best to leave the crooks alone. The street is alive with music, strip shows, street-dancers, and is a carnival scene every night. The streets are washed down early each morning, and by two, the next morning, are covered with trash again. You can have a lot of fun in a night out on Bourbon Street, but one night is enough for most.

Jackson Square with the artist at work painting and musicians playing is a historical spot. The dancers and con men are there too. We enjoyed our stay in New Orleans through March 1999, and will return.

Mobile, Alabama had two hurricanes while we lived there. Sarah announced that we were moving to Arizona. We sold our home in a week, packed and left.

We arrived in Arizona in May 1999. Sarah hired a contractor and built a beautiful home, two bedrooms and a dog room. It was small, but beautiful. We added a separate seven hundred square foot bunk house for guests.

We lived in a twenty-eight foot trailer, from May through November 15, 1999, during construction. We had a good time that summer. It must have been love. We had five dogs that lived with us in the trailer.

The first thing we built was a dog room for the dogs. We built a temporary fence on the back of the lot for a dog run. This was before starting the house.

In Flagstaff, Sarah started showing signs of being manic depressed. She was developing a second identity and the intruder was not welcome. She became overly friendly to the "gay" dog trainer and spent hours on the phone to him on a daily basis.

Footnote: I am angry and hurt — Sarah has told so many lies — a hurt dog bites.

MOBILE SUMMER

Mobile is a very fair city, but in July it is not
Never is it cool in July, it never happens, July is hot — hot — hot

Summer in Mobile does not creep up on you, in July
You are given a sample of it in May and June, and then we cry

It is hot! Yes, it is hot! The blueberries are ripe and so sweet
The lawns and trees are beautiful; the people keep their city neat

True, July is the hottest time of the year
The dog days of summer are clearly here

The outside workers in Mobile suffer the whole month through
The dogs seek the shade, avoid the sun and nap the whole day, too

It is not as hot here as it is in Yuma, Arizona, in July
Needles, California and Death Valley are over 120 degrees, that is high

July, the thermometer rarely exceeds 100 degrees
In winter, we have a few nights that freeze

It is beautiful the whole year, a beautiful city, but when it is not
Never is it cool in July, it never happens, for it is hot — hot — hot!

THUNDER IN MOBILE

I have seen lightning storms in Bangor, Maine
Mobile, Alabama, I have seen the same

The sky billows with flashing light
It flashes between clouds and bolts to the ground left and right

Lightning to the back and to the front at the same time
The hounds roar back as if to rhyme

Flash first, then the bang followed by the hounds roar
The eyes blink wildly and the eardrums are sore

Children cry and women shrink with an unknown fear
Be still all, it is only a Mobile thunderstorm, tomorrow will be clear

The demons, who were here before the storm came
Have been chased to Atlanta, where they will get the same

MOBILE IN JANUARY

We previously reported that July in Mobile was very HOT
January is a beautiful month; a few naked trees, brown grass covers the lot

The robins came through ten days ago and another bunch today
They stay a day or two, brighten up lives with their song and are on their way

The robins seem a little late in flying sought this year
It has been warmer and fall was late; they will all too soon return with spring, I fear

Time is all too short and I hate to see it go by
The robin stops to say hello and never say goodbye

The area is beautiful; if you take the time to look here and there
The beauty is seen by many, but hides from those who neither seek nor care

Beauty does not hide under a rock; beauty sometimes hides in a shadow
The sunshine will, in time, expose beauty to those who gather life's pleasures, and walk slow

Fresno, California had snow last week; grown men made a snowman out in the street
The senior bowl played last week in Mobile; a storm had passed through and it was no treat

Game time, it was seventy, warm, clear and it was sunny
Mobile put its best foot forward for national TV; the players who sought fame and money

Football is, oh, so big in the state of Alabama, where God is still first
The awesome beauty of the ocean port city; the pretty girls and caring people settle the wanders thirst

January is a beautiful time in Mobile; it can be warm or cold
Especially true if you are from Santa Barbara, California, young or old

January 25, 1999

YOU WROTE A BOOK

You wrote a book; it took over two years to do the work of love
Several months later and many rejection letters, you seek help from above

You search for a publisher; someone must be in a great hurry to read your novel; so you think
They after all make all the money, the manuscript you let them read for free; you wink

You seek an agent from New York City; that is where the top agents operate
They make ten percent or more; you expect them to meet you at the gate

You have written your first book, a novel, you seek fame
Slowly you become aware of the fact that it is to be a patient game

The stories you hear start to become clear, be strong, show no fear; they do the driving
The agents don't like new clients; they need to be pampered and praised; you are striving

The war stories you hear add to the worry; that your book may be bad
You had such high expectations that you are down and out, simply sad

This guy took six years before he found a publisher, rewrote the story five times, it was not fun
That lady wrote six books before she found a publisher willing to read one

The publishers are keen to point out that certain famous writers did not publish their first work
That attitude is generally found in a poor class publisher or a real jerk

Seek and you shall find; there are talented people who will read your book
Keep searching; if the book has merit, you will get a fish on the hook

Set the hook firm and strong; they may fight
You will be published if you learn to do it right

January 27, 1999

SUPER BOWL, A BIG DAY

Tomorrow is the SUPER BOWL, A BIG DAY in the United States
A much bigger event than the trial to impeach and toss aside our president ingrate

How in this advanced society can we be so basic, do we only concern our self with today's feast?
We have ethnic killings, starving children, and don't forget their parents; man is not a beast.

We need a rest, a time to hide from the basic ugly truths that be.
Surely there is a better way, we watch grown men sometimes kill each other, but we can't see.

The time requires a searching soul and an inquiring mind to solve the problems of today.
Our minds are truly complex and functions better if given a rest and a time to play.

We of necessity take smiles and laughter as a necessary fuel as well as the food we eat.
Man must always know that behind the clouds, the sun awaits to provide light and heat.

He provides the flowers, the cooling water, our daily bread and requires our praise and thanks.
He does not expect us to be either fools or scowling cranks.

Enjoy the day off for Super Bowl Sunday.
We can always fire the president on Blue Monday.

January 30, 1999

MARDI GRAS IN MOBILE

French for fat Tuesday or Shrove Tuesday is the last day before lent, in Mobile it seems Hell is on the phone.
A time for confession, a time to do penance, but it seems the Roman and Grecian God Backus is being enthroned.

In New Orleans, a murder does not seem out of place during the Mardi Gras celebration.
No one likes it in New Orleans and in Mobile it is a crime that stuns the nation.

Drunks should be arrested when out of place and always when driving a car.
They should watch a twelve-hour TV show that shows drunks in bars, on the street, in auto wreck scenes, drunks on skid row, make them admit the drunks they are.

They should watch these shows and be certified as to being awake and paying attention.
Thirty days in jail or thirty days of twelve hour shows, it would save us money and help more than detention

Those who are guilty of vehicular murder, God alone can help.
Those who lost a friend often cry, imagine how one losing a son or daughter felt.

A killer out to kill an enemy, who discharges a pistol, any gun, in a crowd,
Must be sick, they kill innocent people and care not, they should be executed and no appeal allowed.

The Mardi Gras, in Mobile, is a dangerous place to go and party.
It could be much more fun except for the few drunken smarties.

The parades are early enough so there should be no problem with drunks.
Those few drunks should be arrested and locked up at a drunk rescue mission for lowly skunks.

Release them the morning after; don't worry about booking them
If they show up drunk the next day, lock them up again.

The few who cause trouble are easily spotted; they take away other people's rights
Show the people the beautiful side of Mobile, not the drunks, murders and fights.

Please be nice; Mobile is a beautiful city
Please be nice; the girls are oh, so pretty!

February 6, 1999

October 2001

May 3, 1986 Ike and Sarah were married. They lived together in the following places:

1. Two and a half years in Echo Blue — Lake Wildwood
2. Five years on Buckeye Court — Lake Wildwood
3. 1996 — 1999, Three years in Mobile, Alabama, Colonial Chalet
4. November 1999 — April 15, 2002, Three years in Flagstaff, Arizona

In April 2002, Ike was in Flagstaff and moved back to Santa Barbara. We had lived in Santa Barbara for over four years.

Ike moved to Fresno on October 12, 2002. Table Mountain Casino is in Fresno.

Ike questioned the Joint Tenancy Home purchased on Echo Blue Avenue, in Lake Wildwood. This was a joint purchase. Funds upon sale and collection were deposited in Sarah's Trust account in Mobile, Alabama. Funds from this account purchased and built the home at 119 Kelethon Trail, in Flagstaff, Arizona, and it was community property.

Ike does not and has not disclaimed any interest in the Arizona home. Ike does not know if it is community property and leaves this decision to the courts.

Sarah was stricken with "Bells Palsy" in 2002. We thought she had a stroke. She suffered and was tortured in many ways, not unlike Parkinson's. She had a plastic look on the side of her face. She drooled and one eye had to be taped shut. Her mouth drooped on one side.

Sarah insisted that I care for her and refused outside care. She had more money than she could ever spend. I called her lifelong friend Gay. Help! Gay took charge. She spent two to three weeks out of the next month nursing Sarah.

Sarah was not well, when she threw me out. I could have refused to leave. She, in her demented state, might have killed me. She had tried to throw me over the fence and down a 110-foot drop to the beach below. The Cliffs of Santa Barbara have claimed many victims in the past.

Sarah slugged me. We were out in the backyard and I was attacked by Sarah. She threw a round house right and I was able to jump before the forceful punch landed. It hit me on the shoulder and not the chin. It was a powerful shot and would have downed a lesser man. I was a boxer in former years and I was undefeated. Sarah was a solid 185 pounds and fit.

Shawn saw the punch; Marsha said she did not see it. I did not feel safe with Sarah, but felt the need to watch over her. She might jump over the cliff. She had threatened suicide before.

These thoughts had been my companion for the last three years. Sarah insisted that "she loved me". I believe she did. Her daughters, Marsha and Celeste had told me that they loved me. John deals with reality — never told me he loved me. I believe he did. I loved them all, enjoyed their many visits.

I loved the grandkids too. Marsha referred to me as "that asshole", as we departed the court house. Sarah assaulted me as I started to step out of the courthouse. She spit in my eyes, - brown sticky liquid. It smelled rotten and vile.

I was distraught, hurt, wounded mortally and sad. Why? We had lived together for over twenty years. We had numerous vacation trips (30 to 40), saw many of our states, including Alaska and Hawaii.

We were guests at a formal party at the Annandale County Club. We were acknowledged as the best dance team in the ball and Sarah was told she was the most beautiful. I was a good dancer, at home, on the dance floor, but was far from being handsome. Sarah always will be a beauty to me. Sarah seemed to be attracted to ugly men.

The girl who expelled me from the "White Cliffs of Santa Barbara" vanished and her return is unlikely. The girl left behind is a cruel, countless stranger from the underworld. She will not bring joy or happiness to any she meets.

Attorney Oxford probably told Sarah - You want out, you must move fast. Everyday Clyde stays will cost you as he is living like a king in "The Castle by the Sea"; Support is based upon style and cost to provide quarters, living, food, entertainment, gifts, etc. All you spend is on Clyde. Kick Clyde out fast! Forget love — Sarah you are now talking Big Bucks. You are rich. Clyde is sick and he is old, too. Clyde is also broke. Out fast — Out! You need every penny, Sarah.

Sarah's attorney states that Clyde wasted money Sarah gave him. Clyde gave the list of expenses to them. He lies; I did not waste the money. Sarah lies. I did not throw it away. Sarah gave Peter Belmont $12,000. She spent thousands of dollars calling him on the telephone over the past three years. Sarah told Clyde not to be jealous, because Peter was gay. Sarah's statement that Ike made extraordinary demands for money IS A LIE. Not ONE demand was ever made for money.

Sarah's statement that Ike has symptoms of Parkinson's is wrong. Ike has Parkinson's.

Sarah refused to let Ike drive many times. Sarah would not leave me alone at home. Ike does not drink and has not for many years. Sarah woke up the morning after she hired Attorney Oxford on October 10, 2002 and threw Ike out the next day.

Ike was nowhere to be found was a big lie. In the seven weeks, 24 hours a day I cared for Sarah. I took four or five breaks, one of which was approximately four hours. The others were two hours or less. Sarah had her daughter to call in on emergency and a crew of family and workers. Sarah's daughters took their Hawaii vacations and were aware of my limited ability.

Sarah did not work for 10 of the 17 years we were married. She provided income, on which we lived, by spending over $600,000 of her inheritance property. Mrs. Masterson's will stated: "Sarah to receive the Santa Barbara home clear of all encumbrances."

Sarah stated I wanted to sell my stock to gamble. This statement is a LIE. The stock was sold to pay for my attorneys. re: the divorce. Ike paid $30,000, while Sarah paid $50,000. It should be noted that Clyde ended up breaking even in the stock market. Sarah lost over 25% (probably more) in her stock trading. It was a down market and Clyde did not lose.

Sarah promised Ike $1,000,000 cash and a $5,000 to $6,000 monthly income. Her attorney did not show the Fair Rental Value of Residence or the Rental Property Income.

Ike lived in Sarah's Mother's house for 2 ½ months a year during the 7 ½ years rent-free, following our move to Lake Wildwood. Ike chose to disappear for days at a time. A lie! Ike did not disappear one day. Ike was giving 24 hours a day of his time to Sarah, the dogs and the house. Ike was admitted to emergency at Cottage Hospital, due to a suspected "Heart Attack". He was exhausted and suffered chest pain. Chest pains are serious, for a 69 year old man, with a previous attack and a bundle branch blockage.

Sarah loved me and told the kids she wanted me (Ike) to stay on Sunday, October 6, 2002, five days before Sarah kicked Ike out. It was one day after Sarah had her first meeting with Colin Oxford, Attorney.

Failure to support her is a lie. Ike is a sick man and did his very best, seven days a week.

In summary, Ike gives 100% to survival, 100% to Sarah's care, 100% to marriage. He loves Sarah, but not the greedy power crazy individual she has become. She is a manic depressive and bi-polar. Sarah is sick and not in her right mind.

A few days before she's dismissed, her psychiatrist told Sarah she was not capable of making decisions. The doctor specifically said she was not competent and should not file for divorce.

Ike is a Veteran and entitled to Veteran's Benefits. LIE! Ike never demanded anything. He always asked for Sarah's love and devotion — not a BMW, not a dollar.

Ike gave up his car in 1996 and did little driving at Sarah's request. Sarah told Ike he could not drive, except when she approved.

Sarah received cash gifts, $300,000 gift, auto and jewelry from her mother over the period of June 2, 1986 through October 11, 2002, when she threw Ike out.

The marriage from June 2, 1986 to September 1, 2002 is a period of 18 years. They lived together July 1985 to June 1986.

The so called gambling income was "Several Thousand Dollars" per Sarah and Skip.

Clyde Piatt won three jackpots — per 1099's. It was the first jackpot over $300 Clyde ever won in his life. Clyde's retirement was to be: Sale of business, $300,000; Income from Gunsolley ($135,000. at 7% compounded 1979 to age 65 — 1999, $280,000; Projected retirement fund, $580,000; Yearly income interest, $35,000+. Clyde did not plan to "Hang around until Sarah came into her inheritance. I loved Sarah and as she told her children, on October 6, 2003, she loved Ike and did not want him to go. October 11, 2003, after meeting with Chip on October 10, 2003, her attorney probably told Sarah that she would have to pay support. Her marriage, of over seventeen years to Clyde C. Piatt, a 100% disabled Veteran, who was almost 70 years old, without assets, needed help. At this point in time, love turned to hate.

The love declared on October 6, 2003, was followed by the October 11, 2003 declaration. I hate you, pack and leave now. You have two hours to pack and anything you forget, I will tear up and throw out. In Sarah's hours of need, I did everything I possibly could do. I worked night and day to care for Sarah. Clyde ended up in the emergency ward at Golito Valley Hospital, with chest pain and exhaustion, during the second week after Sarah's operation. Sarah's daughters were aware of the operation, but left for vacation in Hawaii. Sarah was earning $12.50 per hour as a Dental Assistant in 2003.

APPEARANCE OF THE SHREW

She left three years before she said, "You have two hours to pack—get out of here. Anything left will be thrown away."

I said, "I will go; I love you and do not want to go." It was four days before that Sarah's two daughters and her son-in-law, Shawn, asked me to leave… "It would be better for Sarah." Were they really only worried about the money? The three of them assured me that it was in Sarah's best interest. I told them I loved their mother and did not want to go. I reluctantly agreed to go for a few weeks to see if Sarah improved.

Sarah told the three, "She loved me and wanted me to stay". That was just four days before she kicked me out. Sarah had an appointment with her attorney, Colin Oxford, the day before she kicked me out.

I loved her …not the woman she had prepared for her new role in life. Sarah told me, "I am sick and want to be a mean, ugly queen of the White Cliffs of Santa Barbara, living in my castle by the sea." The psychiatrist had diagnosed her as a manic-depressive two weeks before. He told Sarah she was not in her right mind, not to do anything stupid, not to file for divorce. She had become an unknown woman. She had turned into a fat and ugly woman…a complete stranger, a toad. My beauty had disappeared.

The girl I loved was beautiful, loving and caring, as I saw her. I had loved this strange, curious girl, I married. It turned out she had died the year her mother became ill. It was after her mother's attorney had read the will. There was a clause forbidding a change in beneficiaries after Mrs. Masterson turned 75 years of age. The new will also included other changes. A new codicil was signed two months before her death, clearly not legal. Mrs. Masterson was in an alcoholic daze. Sarah's mother called every day, sometimes twice. I answered as Sarah had gone back to work. Mrs. Masterson was out of her mind, legally incompetent. Mrs. Masterson, the Lady in Red from Santa Barbara, changed her will on her deathbed. One and a half million dollars was left to her friend, a Monsignor Priest in Los Angeles. She left the estate administrator over a million dollars in stock. She had left two million dollars to her boyfriend, in the previous will. The codicil had changed that to one million dollars. This was not legal.

Sarah had a lot of friends; she told them I was not able to write anymore, that I was brain dead. She told them "she loved me, but was afraid I would have a claim against her estate."

The writing of this note is without feeling. My love left when Sarah was depressed and the "Ugly Bitch of the White Cliffs of Santa Barbara" appeared. This newcomer was cold, calculating, nasty and a user. Greed had consumed her soul. She had a meeting with her divorce attorney the day before she threw me out. Her parting words were, "You will not get a penny out of me." Her daughter, Michele, and her husband, Shawn, asked me what I thought I was entitled to. I said I was not aware of any "entitlements", but would leave it to the courts. The judge can award anything he decided. He has almost unlimited power per California law.

I was assaulted in that courtroom. Sarah spit in my eyes as I was leaving. It was worse than a camel spit. A brownish, sewer-smelling mouthful was spit in my eyes. As I opened the door of the court, she was yelling, cursing, no class; she attacked me. I was dumb-founded and could not understand Sarah's actions. She laughed and Marsha called me an "asshole." This girl, I had not met before. This stranger tried to push me over the cliff. She threatened me with, "I have the phone number of a hit man and he can take care of you. She told me, "I hope you have brain cancer." She told me "to kill myself". Love had turned her into a shrew. I trust that she does not expect recompense. She is not the one I married. It is the devil trying to take over the "Castle by the Sea". She is a hoax. She is possessed by her mother's ghost. The hoax is not my love; she does not care. My love was a caring, loving fun person who shared. The "Lady in Red" is dead; her spirit haunts the "Castle by the Sea."

The White Cliffs of Santa Barbara, a special, beautiful place to be. March of 1985 she loved me; October 6, 2003 she loved me; October 11, 2003 she ordered me gone.

Tuesday, October 22, 2002

To: Sarah R. Landis
Her Castle by the Sea
Santa Barbara, California

It is 2:51 in the morning and I sleep not
A Senior Citizen in his golden years
The path behind me is cluttered with broken dreams
The never-ending night is without joy — black clouds of death waiting
Parkinson's stalks me. A few seconds of sleep
Then it screams and with a great shake, it wakes me in terror
Terror of the time when he waits to rob me, of everything but life
He must surely hate me
Now, he with a surgeon's help has robbed me of my great love
The love is given freely
And I have not the power to turn away
Yes, He almost killed my love
It was a breast implant and a tummy-tuck operation — a simple procedure
The surgeon left a sponge in her breast
And He was apparently playing golf with the surgeon
I tried to help chase away the pain
Stop the endless stream of horror — puss pouring out of her breast
The endless phone calls with the surgeon on call — lost and unanswering

My love screamed that I was in the way
The beauty is still the same as the day I first met her
She too, is in her "Golden Years"
But her beauty beams from her soul.
Beauty had a pet that day and she stopped by in April 1968
"Dandy Lion" was his name, a thirty-five pound lion cub
They were a beautiful pair.
They matched beauty, spirit, and keen awareness
And a strong lust for life
One had to notice joy that flowed from their endless energy.
The surgeon stole the joy
My love walks bent over
Her mocking eye that won't close
She lives, but with pain and a twisted smile
It would have been kinder of the surgeon
He should have informed my love of his trip
To the old and ancient golf course at St. Andrews, Scotland
He, Mr. Surgeon, should have taught his very competent back up surgeon how to answer a page
My love is still beautiful
Her pain is great
She has been tortured and pain has driven her into a mental ward
She suffers yet
The Bell's palsy, the breakdown, the physical pain leave scars.
She tried to jump off the cliff
The scars may require a discerning eye to see.
One who looks can see
Her beauty and my love for her remain unchanged
Someone gave me the gate — it was not my love
My beauty has gone away
The imposter who is robbing her of joy and love will soon go away
My love for her will remain until "Death" takes me away

May 2002
Dear Marsha, Cookie and all,

I mail this with a troubled heart.
If you will please give them to my one and only love, I date not.

A great pain has consumed me. It will not go away
If I could only wish yesterday's mistakes out and start again.

I realize Parkinson's needs a miracle to be chased away
My love for Sarah remains unchanged.

I love her with every moment of life, awake or sleeping.
I write and will survive.

A large part of me has died.
I wish her cured and happy too.

Love,
Clyde C. Piatt

November 30, 2002
Dear Ginny:

The enclosed are a few personal letters and copies of a few of my attempts to write.

It is a part of my second book. The rewrite of the first book is completed. I do want your opinion as I value your opinion, but the first draft had so many errors, that I did not want you to see it. This was short-sighted on my part. This sample of my work will not be appreciated by Sarah. Beauty and Toad, He must have been very angry when He made me. The enclosed picture is the best picture ever taken by us.

The past six weeks have been my worst days ever. I am trying not to feel sorry for myself. God was tired and found guilty by members of the tribe. I found Him guilty also. The devil is treated better than me.

Sarah used to make fun of my involuntary jerks, facial expressions, saliva dripping, etc. I did not laugh or mention this to my love — I cried inside for her, when she had the same problem and her eye was blank. Sarah was stricken with Bells Palsy.

Ginny, you are a rare friend of Sarah. You are a special friend to this shaky man. You don't pull punches and have been hurt, too. The night you asked me what Sarah was doing, playing post office with the Veterinarian that night many years ago…

Melanie Markusson told me that the moment I left to make a phone call, Sarah disappeared. She was smitten with the caretaker of the fishing cabin and store in Virginia Lakes. She did not cover for Sarah either.

Laura Thompson told me that she was not covering for Sarah. Sarah had told me she was at Laura's for those hours Sarah had disappeared.

It hurt, but I do love her. I did not want to clip her wings, but I was ready to battle the devil to keep her. I will not and cannot share her. Nothing has changed and I am going to give it my best. There is nothing she has done that I cannot forgive:

If she wanted me dead and hired a hit man — I would forgive her.

a. If she fed me poison — I would forgive her.

b. If she had an affair — I would forgive her.

c. If she gave me Parkinson's — I would forgive her.

There is nothing I would not forgive, if she loved me as she attests to. The slate would be polished clean. I have the strength, the will and the great desire to do this.

I beg her to forgive me for not making it clear to her that I would never leave her. It was my way out of our fights, to pack or threaten to leave her. It was a lie. I would have begged to come back. It is true, my first marriage — 21 years — and the marriage breakup was probably my fault. I have never had an affair, since my first date with

Sarah. She is my love — my one and only, forever more. I have never, NEVER had an affair with another man's wife.

With my hands tied, back behind my back, with a sack over my head, with my head on the block — I give the sword to my love.

AMO, AMAS, AMOT, SARAH

THE LADY IN RED

Alas, the "Lady in Red" is dead
Mendacity, she sleeps in her daughter's bed

The White Cliffs of Santa Barbara she rules,
Tenacity, the hangers-on are ghouls

Ghosts, lost souls, a plenty abide
Listen, screams, breaking glass, moans and groans, from inside

Get out fast; go never return
Love lives not here, only spooks that forever burn

Joy and laughter were deposed and put asunder
Chased away by avarice, greed and thunder

Fifty rotten years rule by Scrooge the fool
Now a successor is her tool

Hate, murder, rape and plunder
The "Lady in Red" lives and will never be chased asunder

The White Cliffs will suffer two score and ten
The imposter will leave, the curse passed to the next of kin

December 7, 2002

THE DIAGNOSIS AND PROGRESSION OF SYMPTOMS

I had acquired a twitch in my right hand, thumb and index finger. My eleven year old, step-granddaughter visited us for ten days early May of 1986.

We, the three kids and I were driving from our home in Lake Wildwood to Santa Barbara, California. We were singing songs, telling stories and having a good time on the, 435 mile, journey. Nicole jokingly said, "Your finger is ALIVE!" The index finger and thumb were snapping open and closed, like a telegraph key. Steady and swift, fifty to eighty times a minute.

It was a week before I returned to Lake Wildwood. Sarah had not made the trip, just the three kids and me.

I did not know what was causing the tremor. I had been using a ten key machine for many years and thought it could be the cause. I chose to ignore it and thought it was a "carpal tunnel" problem. I was getting nervous and it was time to address the tremor. I discussed the twitch with my wife, Sarah and we decided I should see a neurologist. Sarah made an appointment with Dr. Sayer, a neurologist, in Sacramento, California, on May 14, 1986.

Dr. Sayer walked into his waiting room, held out his hand, introduced himself and told me to "walk down the hall to his office". He walked behind me. He asked me to "stop in the hall". He told me to "brace myself"; he was going to pull me backward to test my reflexes.

We entered his office and he told Sarah and I to set down. He said, "I had Parkinson's Disease. He said there were no tests he could run to verify it, but he was prescribing the drug Sinemet for me. He said, "If the tremor responded, I had Parkinson's." Nothing much made any sense at the time. The past twenty years have proved his prognosis was correct.

The simple tests and observations by Dr. Sayer, were duplicated by all the doctors. There are other clues and tests; they add up to an uncontestable fact. You have Parkinson's.

I continued to work. We ate out three to five times a week. We traveled and entertained more than most couples.

Sarah never wasted any tears over the disease. She noticed the rapid changes, but seemed to accept them. We were married on May 4, 1986 and moved to Lake Wildwood in 1988. We lived there for 7 ½ years, before moving to Alabama.

Sarah was the kind of a lady who when she dressed up, put her makeup on, she was a beauty. She had the most beautiful brown eyes. When she would turn them on, even the women would touch her to see if she was real. She was beautiful.

They had a formal dance at the Annandale Country Club, in Los Angeles, and as was the custom, we danced every dance. The last dance was over and we were leaving, when a nicely dressed lady told Sarah she was the most beautiful girl there and we were the best dancers there, too. Sarah had been a dancer in Las Vegas when she was seventeen. The attention was normal for Sarah glowed.

Mahlon DeLong, a graduate of Stanford, Harvard Medical School, where he graduated with honors in 1966, is the Chairman of the Emory University School, Dept. of Neurology.

Mahlon DeLong is a biochemist at Emory. He and his wife raised four children.

DeLong states there is no known cure for the over one million people, in the United States, who suffer from Parkinson's disease.

DeLong is credited with the discovery that the overactive affective brain cells. The confusions signals cause the involuntary movement.

Overstimulation, not inactive cells are the problem. Dead cells can of course do nothing.

Overactive cells cause a problem. Overactive cells can be zapped, killed. He reversed the old procedures of pallidotomy. It was dropped in 1962.

Pallidotomy involves the insertion of an electric probe into the brain. The second probe applies heat — which then kills off the defective cells.

All of the thirty plus Neurologists that I have been examined by accept Dr. DeLong's findings. They all say there is no known cure, but the procedure works in 95% of the time and is effective for many years. The procedure is performed only after the other medicines lose their effect. The operation can be repeated.

We need an input of resource dollars to fund our program. We do not need to suffer the terminal Parkinson's. I called Emory when I thought it was time for me, after I stopped my previous operation in San Francisco. My brain was to be operated on in San Francisco. The crown was in place and blood trickled from the four screws inserted to make the crown fixed. I told the Neurologists and Doctors to get it off.

I was overwrought, tired, exhausted, and had lost my faith in them. I had three days without sleep. They had given me written instructions to get a good night's sleep before the surgery. They put me in the same room where one patient had a broken back and later found out, he had a broken leg also.

The Cleveland Clinic, that I referred as the Cleveland Hospital performed the operation for me. My middle name is Cleveland.

It seems that the whole operating team, and the nurses too, would take turns asking me questions in the recovery room. They finally decided to let me sleep. It seems I had told Dr. Rezai, the in charge surgeon, that he was the devil. He did not talk to me. I explained that the guy he talked to was an imposter. I loved the whole crew. I had explained that my system could tolerate no more new drugs. I had taken Sinemet for twenty years and new drugs, pain or narcotics, sent me on a trip. I was out when the other guy called Dr. Ali Rezai a devil. I apologized for the bad judgment.

The patient has a lot of confidence in the team he allowed to: Drill a quarter size hole in the top of his head. Send a hair sized probe into the subthalamic nucleus, between the lower portion of my brain. They moved the probe a micron at a time to locate the electrical problem area. A wire is implanted and attached to a device in the chest.

The patient is awake during the procedure and talks with the surgeon. The million and a half people in the United States, who have Parkinson's, could benefit from the antibiotic minocyclene and creatine. I have taken minocyclene for twenty years and my Parkinson's has not progressed on my left side to date.

Dopamine stills works for me after twenty years, but maybe it is because of the minocyclene. We all react different and further study is required. I feel that we are on the threshold of a big breakthrough in the next two years.

Parkinson's is exploring the use of gene therapy; the insertion of genes to the brain. The genes are inserted by a virus. The process was explored by Ohio State University.

The results showed 25 to 30 % increase in muscle function. The improvement was as high as 65%, in some cases. They will find a way soon. Parkinson sufferers have to play a waiting game, but it will happen. The money for research is being raised; the Government is spending more each year. We will find a cure if God is willing.

DeLONG DISCOVERED A WAY TO TREAT PARKINSON'S

Tony Heffernan, Contributing Writer In Depth: Health-Care Quarterly; July 24, 1998 print edition

Like many college kids, Mahlon DeLong put off taking a course he thought he would detest. So it wasn't until his senior year at Stanford University that the history major signed up for biology. "It was a requirement." It was lucky for the world that Stanford has such a policy. DeLong, now almost 70, became a physician and trailblazing scientist, whose work gave new hope to many of the one million people in the United States who suffer from Parkinson's disease.

DeLong became fascinated with the study of biology in 1961. He was particularly interested in learning about the brain controls human movements. His fascination prompted him to do graduate study in the field.

'WE WERE ASTOUNDED'

Now the chairman of the Emory University School of Medicine's department of neurology, DeLong is renowned in his field. He changed the conventional wisdom about a cause of Parkinson's, a nervous disorder that produces tremors, muscle stiffness and slowness of movement, among other symptoms.

"Mahlon does not accept the conventional wisdom when it doesn't make sense," said Guy McKahnn, chairman of the neurology department at Johns Hopkins School of Medicine in the 1980's, where DeLong made his discovery by experimenting on primates.

"We were astounded," DeLong said.

While working for McKahnn, DeLong figured out that the cause of the erratic movements of Parkinson's sufferers was over-activity on the part of certain brain cells. The conventional wisdom in the scientific community was that these cells were under-active.

The overactive cells send confusing signals to other parts of the body. Over stimulation, not inactive cells are the problem. A Parkinson's sufferer may want his arm to be still, but the faulty signals may cause the limb to move uncontrollably.

The difference between finding that the cells were over-stimulated rather than the opposite is highly significant because nothing can be done about under-active or inactive cells.

But overactive cells are another matter. They could be demolished. "By destroying them, we could abolish the symptoms of Parkinson's disease in animal models," DeLong said. The primates were made to be "Parkinsonian" by giving them chemicals.

OLD PROCEDURE REVIVED

DeLong acted on his discovery by reviving and improving an old surgical procedure, pallidotomy, which had been abandoned in the 1960's as a treatment for Parkinson's. This involves insertion of a microelectrode probe into the brain in order to find a small group of malfunctioning cells, a cluster that measures about 6 millimeters in diameter. Once found, this group of cells is destroyed by using a second probe that permits heat to be applied to small areas of the brain. This lesioning procedure is not a cure, but gives patients an almost immediate return to near-normal lives, which lasts for several years.

Since performing his first operation in 1992 on a human patient, DeLong and his Emory team have performed 300 of the procedures with a 95 percent success rate, he said. The procedure takes three hours, during which the patient is awake.

"Pallidotomy … is now offering hope to thousands of persons, young and old, with Parkinson's," wrote Michael M.E. Johns, executive vice president of health affairs at Emory's Robert W. Woodruff Health Sciences Center, when nominating DeLong for the award.

MUHAMMAD ALI TREATED

DeLong has gained some fame by treating for Muhammad Ail, the retired heavyweight boxing champion. Other physicians who have observed Ali contend that he has Parkinson's "syndrome," not the disease itself. They say his abnormal movements may stem from the punches he received, during his lengthy career, in the ring. He was the champion for many years and gave much more than he received.

DeLong disputed this. "He truly has Parkinson's Disease," the ex-champ's doctor said. DeLong said he has discussed with Ali undergoing a pallidotomy, but the former fighter declines. "He is very independent and he has his own ideas," DeLong said. "He sees it as something to overcome and not something to overcome him." In any case, DeLong said, Ali is still quite mobile, and his medication still helps him. "He's doing so well, relatively speaking, on his own," DeLong said.

Candidates for a pallidotomy are usually patients whose medication is failing them. The reason the procedure was abandoned more than three decades ago was the discovery of an anti-Parkinson drug, Levdopa.

Parkinson's disease starts with the brain's losing the cells that produce a chemical, dopamine. The disappearance of dopamine, in turn, causes other cells to start overacting, and they send aberrant signals to other parts of the body. The result may be that a person wanting to start walking may simply become "frozen," or forced to stand still for several minutes. Or an arm might shake uncontrollably.

The over-stimulating cells are the ones that are eradicated by a pallidotomy.

Levdopa is an artificial form of dopamine, and it relieves Parkinson's symptoms significantly, and, in some cases, totally. But for some reason, after five to ten years, the drug's benefits not only wear off, but the medication begins to cause undesirable side effects, such as the sudden grabbing of something or someone.

At that stage, the patient is probably ready for a pallidotomy. Although this is not a cure, it gives about four to six years of relief for patients who continue to take their medication.

RESEARCH TOOK 20 YEARS

DeLong said he did not come up with his overactive cell conclusion overnight. It took him 20 years of research to get to that point. After completing his internship at Boston City Hospital in 1968, he joined the National Institute of Mental Health, where he stayed five years as a researcher. There, DeLong began to study a part of the brain called the basal ganglia simply because so little was known about it.

In 1988, toward the end of his 15-year stint at Johns Hopkins, he would determine that overactive cells in the basal ganglia were causing Parkinson's symptoms in primates. "That was basic science at its best, to understand motor control," said Donald Price, a neurology professor at Johns Hopkins who worked with DeLong.

In September 1990, DeLong co-published an article on pallidotomy findings in a medical journal, Science, which is credited with igniting the resurgence of interest in the procedure as a Parkinson's treatment.

TEACHER INFLUENCED HIM

While doing graduate work at Stanford in 1961 and 1962, DeLong said, he was influenced by one of his teachers, Donald Kennedy, a distinguished biologist. In 1980, Kennedy become Stanford's president and held that position for 12 years. Kennedy inspired him to become a physician and researcher, DeLong said. "Don Kennedy told me, 'go east young man,'" DeLong recalled. So, the Jefferson, Iowa, native headed for Harvard Medical School, from which he graduated, with honors, in 1966.

DeLong said he was lured away from Johns Hopkins by Emory in 1990 to direct its medical school's neurology department because the university had made a substantial commitment to fund research in his field.

"Emory always made major investments for a strong clinical presence," he said. In the last 20 years, it has made major investments in developing the research arm."

The task ahead is to try to find even better treatments not only for Parkinson's, but for other neurological disorders such as Alzheimer's and dystonia, DeLong said. Dystonia's symptoms are similar to Parkinson's disease, but dystonia attacks children far more often. It also can be treated by the pallidotomy procedure. But the technique is not a cure, and more research needs to be done to improve the outcomes of patient's treatments, DeLong said. "It's not permanent," DeLong said. "'It's progress."

The attached letters to Dr. Mahlon R. DeLong tell the story of my war with Parkinson's. The battle has been an on-going one. The pain and suffering increase each day.

Report to Dr. DeLong

Time for report number three, I feel more like me, it is so much easier to smile
Sleep is steady at six to seven hours nightly, no longer is it up and down with the sun dial

The team now consists of the new players, Tasmar and Paxil
Old players Sinemet and Permax still play; this report is factual

I try to stick with the script, as set up by the manager Dr. DeLong
On a few mornings I slept late, was late taking my first pills, up and singing a happy song

The wife demands that I stick to the script and be a fulltime player
For years, I had lost the desire to sing, to eat, to live and forgot my prayers

In life, I am now a full time player and a part time prayer, too
Your program is great, the shakes are still with me mornings, but you chased away the blues

My wife and I thank you and your wonderful staff
For returning the long lost ability to laugh

July 26, 1998

Clyde C. Piatt5-29-01

Dr. DeLong
EMORY UNIVERSITY

Clyde, as of May 29, 2001, please follow the prescribed dosage below for Mirapex.

Plan 1 - from June 1 through June 22, 2001: 0.125 mg, 3 times a day - 7:00 a.m., noon, and 5:00 p.m. Plan 2 - from June 23 through July 6, 2001: 0.25 mg3 times a day - 7:00 a.m., noon, and 5:00 p.m.

Plan 3 — from July 7 through July 17, 2001: 0.375mg, 3 times a day.

Plan 4 — from July 18 through July 31, 2001: 0.5 mg, 3 times a day for a total of 1.5 mg per day.

Plan 5 — from August 1 through August 11, 2001: 0.75 mg, 3 times per day.

Plan 6 — from August 12, 2001 forward: 1 mg, 3 times per day.

Note: You can increase mg. slower if you don't need an increase.

Clyde C. Piatt, C.P.A.
1054 Chalet Dr. W.
Mobile, Alabama 36608-3613

August 8, 1998

Dr. Mahlon R. DeLong
Emory University School of Medicine
Chairman, Section of Neurology
1365 Clifton Road N.E.
Atlanta, Georgia 30322

Dear Dr. DeLong:

The program you scheduled for me is working far better than I thought possible. It is two months and I feel like I did twenty years ago. I had given up feeling joy; my mind was clouded from noon on each day. My wife had about given up too. My Parkinson's had been diagnosed ten years earlier. I obviously had Parkinson's ten years before I knew what it was. A CPA who was a tax expert, I experienced many of the classic signs. My last few years of work, I was at war with myself. In this office when no one was around, I would force myself to the point that I stood up, raised both of my arms and screamed. Those years were dark and terror was my companion.

Work was both necessary and the second most important part of my life. My wife and family remained first when the neurologist told my wife and me that he was sure I had Parkinson's. I know fear. My first question was "Will my mind remain clear?" Next, "Will I be able to continue my work?" I planned on working my whole life.

He assured us that with medication I could continue for many years. My wife's first question was there any side effects from the medication. He said there were none from Sinement.

Dr. DeLong, when we first met, I was and had been taking the following medications: Sinement 25/250 every 3 hours, 6 times a day and Permax 1 tablet 3 times a day

I had lost the desire to smile and found it difficult to laugh at life's funniest twists. I felt like crying at times and would have if I were not raised by parents who said "men don't cry". I was blue. You and your fine staff prescribed the following: Sinement 25/100, 1 ½ tablets every 3 hours — 7 A.M. until 7 P.M. (7 ½ tablets daily); Tasmar 100, 7 A.M., 1 P.M., 7 P.M.; Sinement CR 25/100, 10 P.M., 1 tablet daily; Paxil 20, 7 A.M. daily (delay 3 weeks); Permax, 1 ½ tablets 10 A.M., 4 P.M.,10 P.M.

It is a minor miracle to me, but overnight my mind cleared. I began to smile again. I easily could laugh and I could sleep. I have a higher energy level and, like the straw man, I feel that I have a brain. I have not suffered any grandiose feelings, nor have I suffered hallucinations and no nightmares. I do not smile as readily as in my youth, do not laugh as hardily, but few do at age 64.

I trust this medication will continue to be effective. Friends have expressed delight to see my return to the real world. With a smile on my face, I thank you and your great staff. My wife and family thank you, too.

Very truly yours,
Clyde C. Piatt

October 25, 1998

Dr. Mahlon R. DeLong
Emory University School of Medicine
Chairman Section of Neurology
1365 Clifton Road NE
Atlanta, Georgia 30322

Dear Dr. DeLong:

The last report you received from me was dated August 8, 1998. I have done better than I thought possible in June 1998. There have been seven or eight times when I have reverted back to the:

Walk leaning forward on toes — feels like I could fall; Wife reports that I hved glassy eyes; Mind is cloudy; Difficulty with words and speaking in general; Seems to be worse with stress of computer and upset at times; Rest one to two hours and I am better.

I do feel and operate much better than before June 1998 when you changed my medication. It seems that I am complaining, but that is not the case. It is difficult to complain when life is so much better than last year. Stick with the facts.

The level of the complaints the past two months is very small. The level allowed me to be creative, to feel challenged and be productive. I wrote a number of stories and finished a book.

Again, with a smile on my face, I thank you and your great staff. My wife and family thank you.

Very truly yours,

Clyde C. Piatt

EMORY UNIVERSITY SCHOOL OF MEDICINE
Department of Neurology

The Robert W. Woodruff Health Sciences Center
Emory University School of Medicine
Woodruff Memorial Research Building
1639 Pierce Drive, Suite 6000
Atlanta, Georgia 30322
Tel.404-727-3818
Fax 404-727-3157

An equal opportunity, Affirmative Action University

December 18, 2002

Re:Clyde C. Piatt
911 Kletha Trail
Flagstaff, Arizona 86001
DOB: 02/11/1934

Dear Sir or Madam:

The above named patient, Clyde C. Piatt, was initially seen in the Department of Neurology, The Emory Clinic, on June 16, 1998, for evaluation of Parkinson's disease.

Mr. Piatt noted that his first parkinsonian symptoms date back to 1986, when he developed right hand tremor. He was diagnosed with Parkinson's disease several years later, and soon thereafter developed gait difficulty and fine motor problems, including handwriting changes. He was placed on the medications Sinemet and Eldepryl and demonstrated a good response; however, the Sinemet caused nausea. His course since then was marked by a gradual deterioration.

At the time of Mr. Piatt's initial visit to the Emory Clinic, it was determined that he had idiopathic Parkinson's disease, primarily affecting the right side, and tremor predominant. In addition, he demonstrated depression and anxiety and possible right side radiculopathy.

When Mr. Piatt returned to the Emory Clinic on October 27, 1998, it was noted that he had moderate to sever tremor of the right arm, mild tremor of the left arm, mild to moderate tremor of the right leg, and mild facial tremor. In addition, he demonstrated moderate bradykinesia, moderate to severe impairment of right foot agility, and mildly stooped posture.

When he was last seen at the Emory Clinic on May 29, 2001, Mr. Piatt continued to demonstrate worsening parkinsonian symptoms, primarily on the right side. In addition to the tremor, he had developed dystonia of the feet and significant dyskinesias when "on" his anti-Parkinson's medication. He had also developed some cognitive dysfunction.

At that time, an adjustment in his anti-Parkinson's medication was recommended. His medications at that time were Sinemet 25/100, Sinemet CR 25/100, Amantadine, Mirapex, Tasmar, and Prozac.

Mr. Piatt has been scheduled to return to the Emory Clinic on February 25, 2003.

As a result of his Parkinson's disease, Mr. Piatt is considered to be totally disabled. Parkinson's disease is a progressive degenerative neurological disorder; therefore, his prognosis is poor.

If there are any questions or if we may be of additional assistance to you, please feel free to contact our program coordinator, James R. Stanton, at 404-712-8485

Thank you very much for your cooperation and assistance.

Sincerely,

Mahlon R. DeLong, M.D.
Professor and Chairman
Department of Neurology

PROSTATE CANCER

March 2003, I was operated on for a prostate problem. They found cancer. I have suffered ever since I had Iodine 125 seeds implanted eight months ago. The cancer is probably gone and I anticipate the disappearance of the radiation sickness.

My second marriage ended October 14, 2002. My wife had a breakdown and was diagnosed as "manic depressed", a bipolar problem. She kicked me out and gave me two hours to pack. I loved her and love her still, but she has gone away. A demon has claimed her body and soul.

I detest the use of "I", I am a fighter and Social Security is an absolute God-send program and must be saved. We cannot have the average American providing his own retirement. The small investor loses money in the stock market. Investing for retirement requires great skill. We have the need to provide a minimum retirement for them.

September 16, 2004 - Appointment with Dr. Samir Arora

A brief history of recent events: I moved to Alabama in 1997. I then noticed an infection in 1998. When living in Fresno, I noticed movement in toes, when hot.

Can we check for cause with ultra sound, by sonar, sound waves or x-ray? Will anything show up on MRI? I am tired of being "left in the dark" and want it resolved. I will pay cash for the tests! I will go to a Psychiatrist.

DEEP BRAIN OPERATION (# 1)

They started the operation in San Francisco, California on March 12, 2004. I was prepped, had the box device screwed on my head and the neurosurgeon was prepared to operate. He drew his map on my shaved head. The purple lines were gross.

They ran me through many tests, mental and physical, over the two months prior. They left me with doubts and, at the last minute I refused and told them to remove the cage. I lost my faith in their work.

The staff had promised me a neurologist would be available during my stay in the hospital. The medical staff available did not know what problems would be to a Parkinson's patient who had been taking Sinemet for eighteen years. The Doctors were not available and could not be reached by phone.

I took Sinemet every hour including sleep hours. I woke up shaking every night, sometimes so violently that I struggled to get out of bed and drag myself around the apartment until the Sinemet took effect - a hellacious struggle. I had no idea of the withdrawal pain, but anticipated a rough time. I was to go "cold turkey". The urge to pass water was further torture. It was not possible until the Sinemet took effect. I had no idea of the withdrawal pain, but anticipated a rough time. No medications allowed after midnight. No aspirin or pain pills either.

Their detailed instructions said, "I should be well-rested for the operation." The hospital room was shared with three trauma patients.

Patient number one was an accident victim with a broken neck. He screamed in pain for three hours. They brought in ex-ray machines to take ex-rays. They found out he also had a broken leg. He was not able to answer any questions, did not know his own name nor did he know where he was. He answered all questions with a "Yeah".

Question 1: Do you know your name? Answer: "Yeah"

Question 2: What is your name? Answer: "Yeah"

Question 3: Do you know the date? Answer: "Yeah"

He suffered the three hours and he was my roommate.

Patient number two had a double hip replacement. He moaned a lot, but was aware of his surroundings.

I was not given a pain pill, Sinemet, or water after midnight in preparation for the surgery. I was concerned and anxious, mostly over the possible withdrawal problems associated with Sinemet.

The instructions told me to be well rested. With three trauma patients sharing the room, I did not sleep. As a result of the drug, I got up five or six times a night to pass water. I could not go and developed a painful retention of urine. I asked for the doctor; the resident doctor came and I requested she call the neurologist. She was asked to insert a catheter. She refused and said, "The neurologist was not available."

I argued with the doctor and demanded that she drain the urine. I told her I was afraid of a system shut down. The withdrawal effects of eighteen years of Sinemet were not known. The young, intelligent, attractive, recent graduate of San Francisco Medical School, finally agreed to insert a drain. She drew off over 1200 cc of urine and blew up my prostate. She apologized that morning. The nurse, on duty, said I was right. It was VICTORY! The prostrate was operated on five days later at St. Agnes Hospital.

I suffer from leg cramps and this night they were horrid. No pain pills as the surgery was to be performed and no medications were allowed after midnight.

My son, Cameron and two of my school friends, from the fourth grade, arrived early, the morning of the operation. I am suffering horrible leg cramps. The left leg convulsed every 44 seconds. Both legs would knot up hard with cramps. My son and school chums took turns massaging the knotted legs.

I somehow managed to make it to the operating section and the department coordinator showed up at 7:00 a.m., never once having checked during the night. I was concerned as they were not being honest with me. They promised to be available, on call.

"Be rested for the surgery." …I was a miserable patient, exhausted and weary. There were many tests to be performed prior to the surgery. They drained all residual strength out of me. I was beat. I had yet to listen to the loud noises that they bombarded my brain with before surgery. The surgery was to be done that morning early. It was 10:00 before I threw in the towel.

I expected a sterile, white room for brain surgery. The staff had not shown me the room prior. I would have dropped out far sooner, not at the last minute. The team Doctors had given me little more than hello and good-bye prior to this day.

They never introduced me to the previous patients. I met two and introduced myself. They did not perceive my interest or question. They appeared demented and confused. I was desperate to try, not wanting to die or be disabled

It took me a long time to admit, but I was ill, exhausted, weary and distraught. No breakfast, tests and a doctor who did not give me lunch, until I demanded it. "Be rested, they told the patient." I was tested from 7:00 a.m. until 2:00 p.m. The lack of caring made me question their motives.

I explained to the Doctor, that without several meals each day, I lost my ability to speak, solve problems or walk. In effect, I told her I would be unable to take any I.Q. test. They wanted my tests to show an improvement after the operation. Did they want me to appear dumb before the operation?

I demanded lunch around 2:00 p.m. I was tired and he said over and over, "Just a few more questions and we are through. He was lying.

A simple true or false, multiple-choice questionnaire is available to test one's I. Q. To say, I am average is a slap in the face for my "Golden Years.

My son, Cameron had a similar experience. He was in the second grade and his lady teacher had slugged him. I called her as soon as he came home and told me. I called a neighbor, a classmate, who was there and verified the facts; his story was the same as Cameron. I called the school Principal and he said, "Cameron's story was probably true." He had been having trouble with her.

I called the teacher and she denied hitting my son. I told her good-bye, and she wanted to discuss the matter. I told her of my findings, that she was lying, and I was wasting my time talking to her.

I had asked Cameron, before, if he wanted to charge the teacher. He said he was smarting off and was wrong. He volunteered to and did stay. I met with the teacher and she apologized. The stress was getting to her. I asked the teacher to evaluate Cameron. She said Cameron was just an average student. The school tested him the next year and he tested as a "gifted" person should.

While in high school, Cameron was admitted to college. He had an "A" average, in college, while a high school student. I, also, have been tested many times and test high. I was in group one in the Armed Forces and tested higher than anyone else in the regiment in math, number one out of 3,000 men.

Testing people like to make their own rules and do not rely on fair testing sometimes. They seek the powers of God and not the truth, except as they see it.

I walked out on the operation, after prep screwing in the crown on my head, at 10:00 in the morning.

June 21, 2004

The surgery was cancelled, per my instructions, at 10:30 in the morning, in San Francisco, California.

"CLINICAL INDICATIONS: The patient is a 70-year old gentleman with medically refractory Parkinson's disease who consented to enrollment in the cooperative studies protocol 468, and presents today for elective deep brain stimulator implantation. The patient was counseled as to the risks and alternatives of the procedure, as well as the steps of the procedure itself. The patient consented to surgical intervention.

DESCRIPTION OF THE PROCEDURE: The patient was identified in the preoperative area and given 1 mg of Versed, per the Anesthesia service for frame placement. The Leksell stereo tactic frame was placed without difficulty, using 1% Epinephrine without Lidocaine at the pin sites for local analgesia. Following this, the patient was taken to MRI and underwent MR imaging per the usual protocol for stereo tactic targeting. The patient was then taken to the preoperative area and then to the operating room. He was transferred to the operating table and before any sedation or procedures were initiated, the patient immediately began to complain of a number of things. He stated that he felt like he did not get enough sleep the evening previously and felt that he was too fatigued to tolerate the surgery. Moreover, he complained the irritation and aggravation from the various monitoring devices that were attached to him, including routine monitoring devices such as EKG leads and pulse oximetry device. He was awake, oriented x 3 and appropriate during this time. He stated in no uncertain terms that he did not wish to proceed with surgery at this time. The patient was immediately placed back on the preoperative gurney and was taken to the preoperative area. The patient was engaged in further discussions, and he continued to maintain his desire not to proceed with surgery today. The surgery was canceled before any invasive procedures were performed. The patient's family was brought to the preoperative area and the situation was discussed. The patient will be discharged home per his wishes."

THE FIGHT

ARTICLES, OBSERVATIONS AND TREATMENT

SCIENCE Every Tuesday: Discoveries, breakthroughs, and trends

News that Michael J. Fox has Parkinson's is a grim reminder that a disease with no cure afflicts 1 million Americans. But a breakthrough procedure is giving some sufferers hope for a more normal life in the late stages. Its biggest impact likely will be felt by young patients, such as Fox, 37, who was diagnosed in 1991. Fox had a different procedure, called a thalamotomy, earlier this year that relieved his worst tremors.

A FANTASTIC VOYAGE TO SOOTHE CEREBRAL CHAOS

By Robert Davis Printed in USA TODAY, Tuesday, December 1, 1998

The neurosurgeon pushes a probe no wider than a human hair slightly farther into his patient's brain, stops and listens.

Ali Rezai is using the same kind of computer-aided navigation that pilots use to find a runway in fog. Now, high tech takes a back seat as he relies on his ear to find the very cells in the subthalamic nucleus that are torturing Naomi Friedland, 61, a retired New York City schoolteacher who suffers from Parkinson's disease.

Speakers fill the operating room with the sounds of electrical activity deep inside her head. To the untrained ear, it's just static.

But as Rezai closes in on the trouble spot, he hears the overactive troublemakers: "Vroom, vroom."

This electrical storm is at the root of Friedland's uncontrollable shaking. This neurologic chaos has robbed her of her life. She can't eat or write or dress herself. "I can't do anything, really," she says.

Rezai is poised to rescue her. His success during this test case may affect aging baby boomers destined for their own battle with Parkinson's, which strikes one out of every 100 people over age 65. Though the disease is most common in the elderly, it can strike younger people. Of those diagnosed with Parkinson's, 5 percent are under age 40, including actor, Michael J. Fox, 37. He revealed his Parkinson's battle last week.

There is no cure for the disease, and doctors can't stop it from destroying the brain.

But scientific advancements in computer-aided medicine have helped surgeons find a new way to block the disease's confusing brain signals. Friedland is part of a clinical trial that is measuring the effectiveness of bilateral subthalamic nucleus stimulation, which doctors say is the biggest breakthrough in the Parkinson's fight in 40 years.

Its young patients like Fox who stand to benefit most from the procedure, says Abraham Lieberman, medical director of the National Parkinson Foundation.

"For the younger patients, this will represent something dramatic," he says. "What is accomplished by stimulating this area is very remarkable."

Using the most detailed computer-aided brain imaging possible, Rezai, of New York's Hospital for Joint Diseases, has positioned his probe in the neighborhood of Friedland's trouble. The neurosurgeon knows he's in the right spot when Friedland suddenly stops shaking.

BURSTS OF ENERGY

At that spot he implants a probe, connects it to a pacemaker-like device in her chest and repeats the process on the other side. When turned on days later, these probes deliver bursts of energy that interfere with the diseased brain's chaotic signals.

The result is dramatic: Friedland's hands are calm and her medicine works again.

"To me, Dr. Rezai is a god," Friedland says.

"The improvement is miraculous," says her friend and support-giver, Resah Nagi.

Others agree.

"This looks very, very promising for people with very advanced disease," says Cheryl Waters, associate professor of neurology at the University of Southern California. She predicts the procedure will eventually be used across the nation.

But today, the surgery is still experimental and people like Friedland can have it done only if they are willing to be studied for several years.

The Food and Drug Administration will consider Friedland and others when it decides whether to approve the procedure, which costs about $50,000. FDA approval, expected within two years, is often needed before insurance will cover new treatments.

The FDA won't discuss such trials during the approval process, citing proprietary concerns of manufacturers. But elsewhere, clinical results are encouraging.

Doctors in France and Canada reported good results in a two-year study published in the Oct. 15 issue of The New England Journal of Medicine. That study showed the stimulation improves all motor manifestations of Parkinson's and significantly decreases the medication that patients need.

"The results are very dramatic," says Rezai, one of the first surgeons to perform the procedure in the USA. "This is a very significant advance."

Anything that helps advanced Parkinson's patients is welcome. There are 1 million people in the USA with the devastating disease.

Why Parkinson's begins to destroy brain cells is not fully understood. And doctors can do little but try to help patients function as the disease continues to destroy the brain.

CHEMICAL MESSENGER

The primary Parkinson's treatment is the drug dopamine, a chemical messenger that is created by healthy brains. The lack of dopamine causes frozen facial expressions, muscle tremors, slowed movements, still limbs and trouble walking and maintaining balance. By giving dopamine, doctors can reduce these effects. But over time, the drug becomes less and less effective.

"I've had Parkinson's for 15 years, and the first 10 were really a breeze, I must say," Friedland says. "My medication controlled the shaking. But the 11th, 12th, and 13th year, the medicine began to wane."

Eventually, the chemical imbalance in her brain left her either suffering the effects of Parkinson's or the side effects of the drug, which include exaggerated movements she calls "spastic."

The disease doesn't kill, so it often leaves people twisting at the end of their psychological rope for years after standard treatments have failed.

"They have no life," says Andrea Smith of the Hospital for Joint Diseases in New York. "One man who couldn't use his arms said that when his wife left the house, he had to put his face down in a bowl and eat like a dog. He said after a while you just don't want to go on like that. A lot of them say they wish they would just die."

Surgeons have tried to help Parkinson's patients over the years by intentionally damaging cells in other trouble areas. By damaging the brain tissue that carries chaotic signals, surgeons disrupt the disease's electrical activity.

But these techniques, thalamotomy and pallidotomy, don't help all of the symptoms and can have major side effects.

Surgeons also are transplanting fetal tissue into the brains of Parkinson's patients. This tissue often grows new, healthier brain cells, but progress can be slow and the side effects of transplants can cause new problems for patients.

None of these surgical procedures allows Parkinson's patients to reduce their medication levels dramatically.

But doctors have found that by sending pulses of electricity into the olive-sized subthalamic region of the brain, they can disrupt Parkinson's wrath.

The technique is based on a similar procedure called deep brain stimulation that was approved by the FDA in August 1997 to treat tremors.

Using that procedure, doctors silence tremors by sending electric pulses into the thalamus. The technique goes deeper into the brain to an area where all the motor problems caused by Parkinson's can be silenced.

To get to the spot deep in Friedland's head, surgeons mapped a route that would cause the least amount of damage to other parts of her brain.

A hydraulic driver moves the probe at various speeds: fast through the top of her brain and extremely slow as it approaches the target area. Thanks to extensive computer mapping and basic rules of navigation, the surgeons arrive right on target.

'YOUR BRAIN TALKING'

They know they're in the right place because her brain tells them so. Because there are no pain sensors in the brain, Friedland has remained awake during her surgery. When the probe reaches the area of her brain that should drive her left arm, surgeons as her to move it. A new noise fills the operating room as her arm moves.

"We're listening to each individual cell," Rezai says. "They each speak different languages. It's like going from one country to another."

Patrick Kelly, a pioneering neurosurgeon, says the sounds are so distinctive that it's as if the cells "have their names tattooed on their forehead."

"I tell them, 'There is your brain talking to you,'" he says.

But the most dramatic sign that they've found the right spot comes when surgeons reach an area of Friedland's brain that causes the tremors. Suddenly, the shaking stops.

"It's one of the most gratifying surgeries you can do," Kelly says. "You take people who are in a living hell and in five minutes you change their life. There are very few surgeries where you get that kind of satisfaction."

The attached letter is from the Cleveland Clinic. The procedure and filing requests are shown in plain English. I was operated on in March of 2007, at the Cleveland Clinic. The team was headed by Dr. Rezai and included other surgeons on his team. They are probably the best team in the world and I would recommend The Cleveland Clinic to all the candidates for the operation. The operation was called Deep Brain

Stimulation. During the operation, they drilled a hole and inserted a very small wire into the brain. The main purpose of the operation was to control the tremor in my hands and legs. The successful operation took about twelve hours between the six or seven hour operation and six hours in recovery. It was a difficult procedure and I was exhausted when it was over.

I told the head surgeon he was a devil while they were performing the operation. I apologized after the operation and apologized to the doctors. I explained that the combination of drugs was too much for me. He was a polished gentleman and a remarkable surgeon. His remarkable staff was members of the operating team. Twenty years of the drug Sinemet did me in.

I am very happy with the results. The team was very close on estimating the outcome of the procedure. Some things like the tremor in my hands and arms vanished and are still gone ten months later.

I have suffered with horrid leg cramps and seizures all of my life. One of first things I noticed was their absence. Before I established my bragging rights, three months later they were back.

It is ten months since the operation and most of my results are still cured. It may be reversed in the next year, it may return tomorrow, but I am happy for today.

I was at the end of my rope and felt that twenty years was long enough to suffer. I consider myself to be a miracle. The team may not be gods, but they do work miracles.

THE CLEVELAND CLINIC FOUNDATION

Dear Patient or Caregiver,

In response to your request for information about Neurosurgery for the treatment of Parkinson's disease, we are pleased to send the enclosed information. If we have not answered all your questions and concerns, or if you are interested in this surgery, please contact us at 1-888-223-6588. In addition, you can access information from our website at http://www.clevelandclinic.org/neuroscience.

Thank you for your inquiry. All the best to you and your family.

Center for Neurological Restoration
9500 Euclid Avenue,
Cleveland, Ohio 44195

Medical & surgical management of movement and other neurological disorders

Ali Rezai, M.D., Co-ChairmanJerrold L. Vitek, M.D., PH.D, Co-Chairman

Nicholas Boulis, M.D.Monique Giroux, M.D.
Jaimie Henderson, M.D.Anwar Ahmed, M.D.
Kenneth Baker, Ph.DScott Cooper, M.D.
Thyagarajan Subramanian, M.D.

DEEP BRAIN STIMULATION (DBS) FOR THE TREATMENT OF PARKINSON'S DISEASE

PACEMAKERS FOR THE BRAIN
WHAT IS DBS?

Deep Brain Stimulation (DBS) is a treatment for some patients with Parkinson's disease and Essential Tremor. Many patients with Parkinson's disease respond well to medications in controlling their symptoms. However despite adjustments in medications, over time, some patients become progressively disabled from their symptoms, obtain less benefit from medications or have significant side effects. Patients with poor quality of life despite taking medications may be candidates for surgery.

DBS is effective in treating a wide range of symptoms, thereby giving patients the chance to improve their quality of life. DBS has been proved to work effectively in controlling the tremor, rigidity, slowness of movement, walking and balance problems associated with Parkinson's disease, while reducing medications.

DBS is as effective as earlier stereo tactic destructive surgeries, but is much safer. With DBS there is no purposeful destruction of brain tissue as in procedures called pallidotomy or thalamotomy and there are fewer long-term complications. DBS has the advantage of being fully reversible and it can be turned off which is not an option with a lesioning or destructive surgery. In addition, the ability to adjust the Stimulator non-invasively with a hand held remote device allows the treatment to be modified according to the unique needs of each patient. DBS allows for maximizing the benefits while minimizing any potential complications. Another potential advantage of stimulation is that it does not preclude patients from receiving other future therapies such as transplantation surgeries in the future.

Beneficial effects of DBS have been proven to last for many years and patients undergoing this surgery over eight years ago are still obtaining good benefits. In general, various studies have shown improvement in the range of 50-70% from DBS for Parkinson's disease. The Food and Drug Administration approved the use of deep brain stimulation on January 14, 2002.

WHAT HAPPENS DURING DBS SURGERY?

Surgical techniques can vary between centers and surgeons. The surgical methods described here are those employed at The Cleveland Clinic Foundation in Cleveland, Ohio. The surgery lasts from 5 — 8 hours and is performed on both sides of the brain to control Parkinson's symptoms on both sides of the body.

During DBS surgery a very thin electrode is implanted in the brain. A lead on the electrode is connected to an impulse generator or "pacemaker", which is then implanted under the skin in the upper chest. DBS exerts its therapeutic effect by delivering tiny electrical impulses to a specific region of the brain. The success of DBS therapy is directly related to the localization of precise surgical targets. These targets are located by using high-resolution stereo tactic imaging and computer-guided surgical navigation, as well as physiological brain mapping.

A team of specialists at the Cleveland Clinic Center for Functional and Restorative Neuroscience, guided by the latest advances in computer-assisted imaging and physiological brain-mapping technology, identify the exact location in the brain where chaotic nerve signals generate tremor, rigidity, slowness of movement and stillness. The team includes a group of expert neurosurgeons, movement disorder neurologists, physiologists, radiologists, neuropsychologists, and nurses that specialize in the treatment of movement disorders.

Since the target location for placement of the electrode is exceptionally small, The Cleveland Clinic has acquired the most sophisticated imaging and recording equipment available for the mapping of the brain.

The procedure begins with a metal halo-like device being attached to the head. The patients then undergo MRI and CT scans of the brain to obtain images and to determine the precise location of the desired target area. Once the target area of the brain has been identified, the skin over that location is anesthetized (similar to the technique used by dentists to numb the mouth when dental work is performed). Through a tiny incision in the skin and bony opening of the skull, a temporary microelectrode is placed into the brain. This temporary microelectrode allows for the precise localization of the target by fine-tuning the initial target seen on MRI and CT images. The patient does not feel any pain sensation during this placement in the brain, because of the unique properties of the brain. The patient is awake during the procedure, allowing the surgical team to record brain activity while the patient moves different parts of his or her body. The patient's movements help to determine where the electrode should be permanently placed. The surgeon eventually replaces the temporary microelectrode with the permanent deep brain stimulation therapeutic lead.

DBS

Once the electrode is implanted in the brain, a wire will connect the electrode to a battery-operated device that sends out electrical impulses to the electrode.

For this part, the patient undergoes general anesthesia. The battery-operated device is implanted under the skin, over the chest, below the collarbone. The wire that connects the electrode to the battery-operated device is tunneled under the skin of the back of the head and neck and under the skin over the front of the chest.

WHAT HAPPENS FOLLOWING DBS SURGERY?

Approximately ten days after surgery the stimulators will be turned on and carefully adjusted to achieve maximum effectiveness. A patient's response to stimulation or medication will change during the first few weeks after surgery and refinements of both the stimulator and drug dosages will be necessary. A family member or caregiver receives instruction on how to monitor and respond to these changes. The patients have a few follow up stimulator adjustment visits should be at the center where the surgery was performed, but later the patient's own physician can adjust both the stimulator and medications. The optimal stimulation parameters tailored for each patient can take from 3 — 6 months.

As with any surgery, the procedure is not entirely risk-free. There is a two to three percent chance (or two to three out of every 100) of brain hemorrhage, which may range in severity with the most severe cases causing a stroke, paralysis, speech impairment or other deficits and the more mild cases causing no significant neurological change. Infections can occur in a small percentage of patients as with any other implantable device. Infections are treated with antibiotics initially and may require the temporary removal of the stimulator in severe cases.

After surgery, many patients enjoy a fuller range of movement and the restoration of many activities daily could not be performed before surgery. Patients are more capable of taking care of themselves, working at their chosen professions, doing hobbies and sports and participating in everyday activities that were impossible or extremely difficult before surgery. Overall, many patients achieve their desire—an improved quality of life.

The battery will run down requiring replacement of the battery-operated device. This may occur every 2 — 5 years depending on how often it is used and how strong the stimulation is.

Here are some questions and answers, which may help you decide if you want to inquire further about possibly being a candidate for Deep Brain Stimulation:

WHO IS A CANDIDATE FOR SURGERY?

Any patient who is not satisfied with his/her level of control; Any patient who exhibits Parkinson's disease which cause a decline in the quality of life; Any patient who has adequately and reasonably tried medications; Any patient who has not had symptoms of dementia.

IS AGE A FACTOR?

This surgery has been successful in treating patients in a range of ages, including those in their seventies. However, each patient should be assessed individually as to his or her stamina and overall health before considering surgery.

WHO PERFORMS THIS PROCEDURE?

The procedure should be performed only at a center that has made the investment and commitment to obtain State-of-the Art equipment and has assembled a multi-disciplinary, experienced team of neurosurgeons, neurologists, neurophysiologists, and neuropsychologists dedicated to the treatment of movement disorders.

HOW WILL THE DOCTORS KNOW WHERE TO PLACE THE ELECTRODES?

The team of specialists at The Cleveland Clinic uses advanced computerized brain imaging as well as microelectrode systems for recording in order to map and target the specific areas of the brain they need to reach.

WHAT ARE THE RISKS?

As with any surgical procedure, there are risks. These are best discussed on an individual basis with the team.

HOW EFFECTIVE IS THE SURGERY?

The vast majority of patients experience a significant improvement of all their symptoms related to Parkinson's disease. Most patients are able to significantly reduce their medications.

HOW LONG WILL I BE IN THE HOSPITAL?

Most patients are in the hospital approximately three days after surgery.

WILL I BE ASLEEP FOR THE PROCEDURE?

The patient remains awake throughout the procedure for implantation of the brain electrode. This allows the team to interact with the patient in testing the effects of the stimulation. Small amounts of local anesthetic are given in sensitive areas. The vast majority of patients experience only minimal discomfort. The patients are placed under general anesthesia for a short time for the placement of the pacemaker device to the chest.

HOW CAN I MAKE AN APPOINTMENT?

Please call 888-223-6588

OSU SCIENTIST'S GENE THERAPY

Technique may aid Parkinson's patients; Small study showed improved muscle function

By Mike Lafferty, The Columbus Dispatch, June 22, 2007

Parkinson's patients showed remarkable improvement after undergoing gene therapy delivered to their brains through a virus, according to a new study.

The technique was pioneered by an Ohio State University scientist and described in the current issue of the British medical journal The Lancet. Patients in the small study improved an average of 25 percent to 30 percent in muscle function. And some patients improved by as much as 65 percent. Parkinson's a chronic, progressive disease affects about 1 million Americans, causing muscle tremors of the hands, arms, legs and jaw. The disease affects speech as well as balance and stability.

Parkinson's disease occurs when a person no longer produces certain neurotransmitters such as dopamine. In patients, one gene in particular, called GAD, fails to promote the manufacture of a neurotransmitter chemical called GABA, which helps keep neurons from firing too much, causing tremors.

Gene therapy involves replacing the broken gene with functioning copies that program cells to make whatever protein or other body chemical is needed.

"It's like a car without brake fluid. This area of the brain goes out of control. We're putting the brake fluid back in," said Dr. Matthew During, a molecular biologist and cancer geneticist at Ohio State and lead author of the paper.

If further tests are successful, During said, the technique could be in use by 2010 to treat a variety of neurological diseases, including Alzheimer's, Huntington's disease, Lou Gehrig's and depression.

"We're even considering obesity," During said.

Jack Warner, a 69 year-old Whitehall resident who hosts and East Side Parkinson's support group, said the disease causes rigidity and shaking.

"I've fallen a couple of times and busted my butt real good," he said. Medication has helped, Warner said, but the disease is beginning to affect his driving.

During and Dr. Michael Kaplitt, of the Weill Cornell Medical College, developed the technique to deliver the genes using a harmless variety of virus. The technique is now widely used.

Genetic material is inserted into a virus, which is used like a Trojan horse to get into cells. Once inside, the genes replicate. In this case, the virus contains the GAD gene.

Kaplitt performed the study at New York Presbyterian Hospital from 2003 to 2005. The therapy was performed on 12 patients who were 50 to 67 years old and had Parkinson's for at least five years.

Each patient received between 3.5 billion and 35 billion virus particles in a small area on one side of the brain.

Improvement began after about three months and has continued, During said. One male patient now rides a bicycle.

In future trials, genes will be placed in both sides of the brain. During said he expects improvement to be even more dramatic. Some of the trials might take place at Ohio State, he said.

Dr. Fredy J. Revilla, a neurologist at the University of Cincinnati Medical Center, said the initial study showed the technique is safe.

"It's interesting that there was some improvement in symptoms. However, these results have to be taken with caution because there was no control group," he said.

"It's a procedure that could have a lot of potential but first there has to be larger study with a control group."

Progress can't come too soon for Ed Nies, of Loveland, Ohio.

"When the drugs are working, good people don't realize I have Parkinson's," he said.

But Nies worries about the future and whether he will end up in a wheelchair. Gene therapy, he said, offers hope to speed scientific progress that seems agonizingly slow.

mlafferty@dispatch.com

ABOUT PARKINSON'S DISEASE

WHAT IS IT?

Parkinson's belongs to a group of conditions called movement disorders. It is a chronic and progressive, meaning its symptoms grow worse and last over time. Some of the common symptoms of Parkinson's are tremors of the hands, legs or jaw; rigidity or stiffness of the limbs and trunk; slowness of movement; and postural instability or impaired balance and coordination.

HOW MANY PEOPLE HAVE IT?

As many as 1 million Americans have Parkinson's Doctors diagnose Parkinson's in about 40,000

Americans each year, and thousands more cases go undetected. Incidence of Parkinson's increases with age, but an estimated 15 percent of cases are diagnosed before a patient is 50.

WHAT ARE THE CAUSES?

As is the case with many neurological disorders, the cause of Parkinson's is not known.

IS IT INHERITED?

Although the vast majority of Parkinson's cases are not directly inherited, researchers have discovered several genes that can cause the disease in a small number of families.

WHAT HAPPENS?

Parkinson's occurs when a group of cells, in an area of the brain called the substantia nigra, begin to malfunction and eventually die. These cells produce a chemical called dopamine, which is a neurotransmitter, or chemical messenger, that regulates the activity of parts of the brain that control movement initiation and coordination. When Parkinson's occurs, these cells begin to die at a faster rate and the amount of dopamine produced in the brain decreases, leaving a person unable to control movement normally.

HOW IS IT TREATED?

There is no known cure for Parkinson's. Physicians treat it with medications that treat the symptoms of the disease. Surgical options, such as deep brain stimulation, might help alleviate a person's symptoms if and when they stop responding favorably to medication.

IS IT FATAL?

Parkinson's is a progressive disorder, and although it is not considered to be fatal, symptoms do worsen over time and make life difficult.

For more information, go to the Parkinson's Disease Foundation Web site at www.pdf.org.

Source: Parkinson's Disease Foundation

Why do we save some work? The trash should be thrown out.

AWAY

The days pass slowly, when you are alone
The nights are bad and you wish she would phone

TV, a place to hide is at best, life's sideshow
One could fly away, if they were a dove or crow

A rich man can always count his money
A Pooh Bear can always search for honey

I don't care to fly and am not a rich man
Steal the honey and suffer the Bee's as you dance the can-can

The day was warm, the first day of summer
Spring flashed by and has gone — a bummer

The azaleas and dogwood are beautiful in their spring blooms
There is much beauty around so why the gloom

This man cries and wishes you home
Man was never meant to live alone

She will be home in a few days — four
I pray she will stay — evermore

I cannot tell my story about Parkinson's without a story about my mother. She gives me strength to this day. When I am low, she gives me the necessary power to go.

WHY MOTHER WHY?

Mother was ill and had at the best a week or two; she died November 1987. It was rough
It was my last visit; I had to leave and mother was eager to go, she had suffered enough

My mind wandered the week I had been at her side; many questions I wanted to ask
Somehow they did not seem so important now, but mother was up to the task

She was in bright spirits, no bitterness or ill will, life for her was over, I miss mother
We always could talk, no fear of being ridiculed, we were friends and I had a great love for her

My cousins came to visit us for the summer in July 1945
Betty was sixteen, Phyllis was fourteen; Betty made skates seem alive

Jim and Ike went skating with them many times that summer
The skating rink had hardwood floors and was above the bowling alley

The girls were both very talented skaters; and we mostly skated fast, we flew
They would practice spins, jumps, throws and a lot of fancy steps, too

The skating was done at night and we liked to go along
Summer days were time to swim and play outside where we belonged

Betty and Phyllis had grown up in the El Centro Valley and it was like the Yuma Valley, hot and fun
They could do anything the boys could do; many times they showed us up but good and they loved the sun

Our favorite swimming holes were along the canals in the valley and the Colorado River Canal
The River Canal took water out of the dam above Yuma; it was mainly for the farmers

All canals operate on the same principle as rivers; water flows downhill
The River Canal had a huge spillway; when the gates were open, the canal would fill

The spillway was 200 yards at the top and 400 yards wide where the concerts sides stopped
The sides were slick and twenty feet high, the water level created an undertow action when it dropped

Mother knew all the good spots as she went swimming with us from the beginning
She had a special talent; she was just one of the gang and loved swimming

She always seemed to have as much fun as we did, never complained about too much sun
That was being a part of the gang, no time to complain when you are having fun

Mom could complain about the heat at home, she did hate the summer here, to Mom summer was a bummer

When Dad was able to, he sent mother to Salinas, California for the summer

This day as a treat to Betty, Phyllis, Jim and I, she took us to the Spillway swimming hole
We swam for over two hours, having a good time; it was time to go.
The sun had taken its toll

Unexpectedly, the gates were opened wide, we were caught in the back current and had to think fast
The back current tried to suck Jim and Ike into the Spillway; they had never done that in the past

We were standing waste deep on the sandy bottom of the canal about 300 yards from the spillway
The current was inch-by inch pulling us back into the concrete tunnel, this was not play

Jim and Ike were both excellent swimmers, were knowledgeable about the canal and not to be put asunder
Ike had won the Yuma County Municipal Pool Swim Race on July 4, 1945 for those twelve and under

We decided that we were running out of time as we were losing inches fast
There was a rock barrier that ran about fifty yards before the concrete walls, a chance, out last

We had an inter-tube and each grabbed a side, we swam with the current towards the rocks
If we did not get to the rocks before the concrete we were in for some shocks

The angle we swam should get us to the rock twenty yards before the wall
We swam as fast as we could and said a little prayer; this was a last call

We were losing ground fast and the rocks were still a long way away
My mind was clear and my thoughts were, if we don't make the rocks what do I do this day

Possible alternative ways out were flying through my mind, I had been here before not long past
We swam at another small spillway where the water was not so fast

I knew the water there forced you towards the bottom of the canal; I knew this well
If you fought the flow you were in trouble, but if you swam with the flow to the bottom, it worked swell

The flow would push you out to the main current and the flow would take you out of danger
If we were sucked into the churning water that was my plan, trouble was no stranger

You had to be able to hold your breath a long time
We had both practiced holding our breath, swimming long distances under water, we did it fine

But we still had a chance to make the rocks; we were strong swimmers and playing it as cool as we could
The rocks were getting closer; the current was getting stronger, make it we should

The rocks were suddenly within reach; Jim and I both grabbed for the rocks they were mossier and slick
We slipped; we tried again, without a second thought, this time we held

We were yelling and celebrating our narrow escape when we looked around, we should have looked before
All the many people, soldiers, adults and kids except one had made it to shore

My cousin, Phyllis was still fighting the current; she was in trouble and alone
The soldiers and grownups were just watching, no one would risk going after her, they had turned to stone

Jim and I ran back to the beach, Mother was shouting instructions to Phyllis
Mother, with a solemn look at me, said "Ike go get her"

I was an eleven-year old kid, given a worldly adventurer; I knew it was serious
Without a second though, I grabbed the inter-tube and walked out towards Phyllis, I was curious

Not one person offered to help; they stood silently by, they did not try
It brought but one question in my mind. Why? I would ask later, now I had other eggs to fry

I had a what if plan in mind and thought I had a chance even if we were sucked into the spillway
Phyllis would probably not make it through the rough water; I would have time to tell her the best way

I was a few feet from her when I told her we had to swim cross current to the rocks; we had a good chance
She was three years older than me, but accepted my decision; I told her to swim like it was the last dance

The distance was about the same as Jim and I had swam earlier; the current was stronger
We were losing ground inch by inch and couldn't wait any longer

I tried to think of how to assist her if we did not make it, but there was no way
I did not think it possible for her to understand what I planned; it might not work anyway

She was a good swimmer; we both held on to the tube and swam as fast as we could
We were closer to the concrete wall than Jim and I had been; to grab the rocks, we had to be good

I told Phyllis to grab with all her might; I would dig in my nails
As happened the first time we could not hold on to the slick rocks;
We had time for one more try; we did not fail

We climbed out a foot before the concrete wall; Phyllis was probably in shock
As for me, I was shook, tired and happy to be safe; there was no one I wanted to sock

As I remember, Mother never discussed the event again; it was as if it never happened; what was it about?
I always wondered what had went on in my Mother's thoughts when she told me to get Phyllis out

I never questioned her, but the thought occurred to me, why had she sent me with all those soldiers standing by?
It was dangerous; grown men doing nothing but watching, why?

Mother was on her last week or two of life, and I asked her why?
Mother said that all through life, when she needed help, I was close by

She knew how dangerous it was, but I had to try
We could not stand there and watch Phyllis cry

We turned to lighter topics, laughed and smiled a lot
I asked her to let the family skeletons loose, tell me her secrets, but a smile was all I got

I had said my goodbye and was prepared for the call I received a few days later; she died
She will be with me always, a special Mother, I cried
September 1, 1998

MISS YOU

Like Dad, you left without a goodbye
I am so sad, but don't want to cry

A single tear ran down my cheek
My eyes clouded and I felt weak

She is with me, clearly in my mind
We played golf, had a great back nine

The score could have been a little lower
Life could have passed a little slower

But who keeps score when you are having fun
Your life at long last had just begun

You were an ace, a hole in one; a part of a great pair
You did not say goodbye; it is not fair

My loss is so real; the pain so great
It appears my heart will surely break

The pair of you may be in Disney Land
Or at a ball game watching the Dodgers home stand

You have a new home on the golf course "evergreen"

A beautiful course as never before seen

A desert course, long and hilly
The morning air, crisp and a little chilly

They smile and laugh as the eagles fly
In my heart, they will never die

One more round, one more ride, Easter with me
You will always be a part of me, until I too, am set free

I ask the Eagle to watch over them and keep score
From his high perch, He said, "He would watch over them forever more".

1987

TODAY BIRTHDAY

Cut, bruised, bloodied and distraught,
It was not by plan or in any way sought.

Sunshine, love and fulfillment was my plan,
For all the yesterdays, I have but written my name in the sand.

I loved and cried, smiled and frowned,
In retrospect, I have been both grasshopper and clown.

The pain in my chest steals a much-needed rest.
The pain is the result of a frustrated man,
Who cannot have lived only to write his name in the sand.

The days past have been much less than cheery,
My hand shakes and I am weary.

Death is today on my mind,
I fear it not, but seek more time.

The sun I seek is somewhere shining,
It is not my destiny to leave life whining.

I dare to be remembered for love and caring,
Life's broken dreams were not due to lack of daring.

A small mark of greatness is what I seek.
What is found, must first be lost, I am not bleak,
And miles to go, before I sleep.

PROGRAM A SMILE

My life was like a ship with a hole in it — sinking
The ever-present smile of youth had gone fishing

A new doctor and a couple of new pills
The smile returned with all the frills

YOUTH HAS GONE

I don't know when or how it left, but it is gone
Youth was to last forever, no, so I was wrong

In my haste to grow up, I lost it
The many players scattered bit by bit

There is still time, but no more of the same
No more fantasies, no time to seek fame

Be one with yourself and your chosen friends
To all you have wronged, make amends

Was youth ever here or was it a dream
Never are yesterdays what they may seem

Live a smile and laughter will find you today
Tomorrow is nowhere to be found, wise men say

Today you are ever young and free
Smile, there is no tomorrow for you or me

July 5, 1998

DOWN AND OUT

Parkinson's is a calculating, demeaning and unwanted guest
Those who it visits are the cursed players at best

Who are the players and who is the prayer?
The caretaker or spouse is the prime player

Is the spouse the one is cursed? Could this be the case?
Are they the responsible party and should they be debased?

I, the Parkie, have been trying to think of a reason why
Am I being punished for some long past sin in days gone by?

Was my late hours and drinking the cause of my plight?
Could have been my wife's problem, because she is ever right?

I know not the reason if there is by chance one or two
It is nothing that my wife did or did not do

Blame is neither due one or the other, but may in truth be Mother
Dad may be guilty or a Grandparent, but not my Brother

The cause is unknown, but it has affected my life
But the one that suffers the most is my wife

I wish it were not in any way the case, but she suffers more

She will not accept defeat and is unbowed by the chore

The road is being paved by researchers and caregivers, who say,
“The ride is not as bad as yesterday and is smoother with each day”

Tomorrow may come a complete cure
Today we need only endure

So we need not evermore be crying the blues
Smile, laugh, you have paid life’s dues

July 5, 1998

A TEAM PLAYER

A new player joined the team today
Paxil, a team player has little to say

He mellowed the team or so it seemed to be
He did his job quietly, no big celebration or jubilee

No nightmares or visions, no loud bangs or songs
We will give Paxil a week to see if he belongs

The team needs new players evermore; it's true
Bring them with smiles, clear minds, too

THE GOLDEN YEARS

Retirement: the so-called Golden Years, gray heads and a bucket of fears.
Many a day you greet with a cheer, a big day planned with nothing to do, the day ends in tears.

Growing old is not, in any way, a graceful walk in the park.
The end of the road, the sun goes down with a flash and it is forever dark.

The body complains that it has been mistreated, proper maintenance neglected,
But that anabolism would, for a great Doctor, go undetected.

Planned retirement perfect, children had left the nest, three pensions should suffice,
Retired, as a young man, under forty, from the Military, then 24 years of Civil Service.

Gray hair; back slightly bent, steady mind and content.
The younger spouse had a few more years before retirement.

It takes so little time to grow old, as the years from young, middle, to old are few.
The ancient and wise owl, when asked the question, "What is a person to do?"

Explained that young people should feather their nest with a life long store of happiness.
Memories are life's greatest and only everlasting measure of success.

Memories are hyacinths stored up by time well spent.
They are rewards for those who lived life every day and are content.

There is not a written guarantee that tells the number of our days.
Work and don't shirk your responsibilities, but memories are best by one who also plays.

Retired on Friday as the story unfolded, no one cried.
We all were shocked and cried the following Monday, the day he died.

July 22, 1998

DR. PHIL

A story starts with a beginning
This story has no ending

It is about a gifted surgeon; the husband of a friend of my wife
My wife and she were not related, but sisters for life

The story, as told, is as I remember and is true
It is about an MD; you would have loved him, too

Dr. Phil was born in Wyoming, about nineteen twenty-four
His Father was of Indian descent, a cattleman who took life as is and never asked for more

Dr. Phil had a brother who was a Veterinarian Doctor and one who studied law
The three brothers were all bright, studied, and worked with no apparent flaw

He spent his younger years working on his Dad's ranch; his Brother's did, too
When not in school, they worked long and hard, as they had to do

Winters are cold in Wyoming; working cattle is hard and in winter cold
Dangerous and satisfying work when you are young and more so when you are old

Ranch life seasoned the Brothers and their Father made them determined and tough
The guidance was good, appreciated, and understood when times were rough

Joy came in a bottomless jar and was shared by the whole family
The jar held food a plenty, friendly spirits, warm home in an Indian family free

Time was not to be wasted, as is the Indian way
Words were not wasted and saved until you had something important to say

We did take time out for play; he loved company and always had a joke to tell
My wife and Dr. Phil laughed and cried over the jokes they both told so well

School and work, work and school and a little time for play
Hunting was a necessary part of the ranch then, and is today

The Brothers were all hunters in their younger years
Dr. Phil, for all his sick patients and creatures, in his heart shed tears

For his life was dedicated to saving life, not destroying it
His skill with a knife was better served in medicine than skinning a rabbit

The Doctor specialized in Urology and was a great surgeon, too
He loved his work; a keen eye and a sharp knife, his hands flew

Young Dr. Phil, when the need be, did many operations for free
Never was a sick man turned away for lack of the fee

He was a most unusual Doctor, a prudent investor, and a good businessman
He was raised on hard work, family responsibility and when needed, to lend a helping hand

The Opera, fine wine, good friends, building, filled his non-working hours
No time to waste, he tasted every hour of every day, be it sunny or showers

The Doctor loved hard work and a construction project was his game
Once he tore into a house, it would never be the same

Dr. Phil's Father was an investor and believed that real estate was the way
The Doctor invested in sound commercial properties not to get rich in a day

The investments were doing as planned and times were good too
A friend in need requested aid, promises he made, many not true

The legal problems resulted in personal suffering, untold sleepless nights for the Doctor and his wife
A warrior, he fought the battle for the rest of his life

He was a competent investor, but the best can be cheated
Dr. Phil could be cheated, but his strong character could never be defeated

He was a warrior, both strong physically and in spirit, a fighter to the end
To his family, patients, friends and to my wife a very special, loving Friend

We enjoyed their company, shared their bountiful table, and drank his fine wine
Many times he chased away the dark storms, for my wife and made her soul shine

Dr. Phil's life was filled with family, friends, and a keen hunger for living
Until the days allotted were gone, caring, sharing, healing the sick, filled all his days of giving

The Dr. Phil still watches over his wife and his spirit is with his Family and Friends
He will be with us until our allotted time ends

He will be with family and friends
Far after the time, their allotted days end

July 30, 1998

August 8, 1998

To You and Your Family and Friends:

Today, I announced that I was writing a book of poems, as did my Great, Great Uncle James Piatt. When I was Baptized, I was listed as James Piatt. Was this a coincidence or was it predestination? James Piatt has a published book of poems and was a Poet long ago.

I have written poems since college days and before. Most were thrown away. Some were written inside my class book and some of these, I have today. In a few cases, I have saved some of my earliest efforts.

Originally, and even today, I write to gain knowledge, use a few difficult words and make the rhyme fit the word, an exercise, at best. It pleases me to write in the simplest terms possible. In truth, the story is better, when it can be told simply.

There are times to be repetitive. A rose is a rose, is a rose, is a rose, is noted. There are times to be retrospect and times to be cute; and miles to go before I sleep, tells the story well.

A loud noise may be a wakeup call. A loud, loud, loud noise may put you to sleep. A cry may be a cry or may be a sob or a yell. Words can be made to say different things.

A ring may be a ring or a ring:

Telephone Ring

Ring in a Tub

Ring in a Tree

Ring you wear

We may be free in spirit, in body, of worries, after divorce, of disease, of lice, etc. But, is

anyone really free? No one, I know, or have met is free.

I don't want to be free. My family and friends, my work, and my God are calling me. They and others, I yearn to know better and to serve better.

These thoughts pass through my mind swiftly and I have tried to record them accurately. I will continue to write, hopefully. It would be a pleasure to be published. I have always dreaded leaving this life after only writing my name in the sand. I desire to leave tracks and most of all to contribute to and not take away from life.

Clyde C. Piatt

FORK IN THE ROAD

You are born without a choice, you may choose when you die
The first choice after you arrive is to yell or to cry

Life sometimes makes a place for you, if you make enough noise
The bold make noise and step on people's toes

If you don't enter this world yelling, you get a sharp slap
Smart babies enter yelling, like a turpentine cat

So you see, there is a time to cry and a time to yell
Either way you choose, you must develop your method well

If you fake it and are caught, you are through
No one respects a faker, even if they are fakers, too

You may choose to play the game of life fair
No cheating or cutting corners, you will be a square

Many will take you for a fool and think you are weak
If you are strong, you may make it, only the weak cheat

A part time cheat or one who cheats, only once is a crook
A part time crook is a crook, in no way is a Queen a Rook

You may be bad or good, as it is understood, or some of each
There are various shades one changes, as does a ripening peach

The peach goes from green, to golden yellow, to rotten
Man is born a precious baby and is soon old and forgotten

There are as many forks in the road, as there are branches in a tree
Don't yell until someone steps on your toes, if they are bigger, let them be

Don't be the master of your ship or captain of your soul
Let God run both and make peace and happiness your goal

Tell the truth, live with the truth and be as good as you can
God is perfect, but he did not make a perfect man
August 3, 1998

WRITERS' BLOCK

I remember the first year I opened an office as a CPA in Goleta, California, one of my first appointments, a young lady asked me, "If I was a real CPA".

When I was 27 years old my younger brother and I went into a bar and ordered a drink. He was ten years younger than I. He ordered a scotch and water. I ordered a bourbon and water. The bartender asked me for identification, but not my brother.

Sometime in the early 1970's people started noticing that I was looking older. I aged twenty years in ten. It was Parkinson's, one of the early signs that went on for years. Looking back, I can now recognize the signs.

My face acquired a plastic look and my smile left. I was not happy. I started to lift my right arm with the elbow extended. My right arm gradually quit swinging when I walked. My right foot cramped. These signs were lost to me.

They progressed slowly and over a period of seven or eight years. In 1987, I got the first really noticeable sign. My thumb and right index finger started to shake. The first tremor occurred when I was under stress or over tired.

There were other signs. I played chess with a long time friend and he started winning. He noticed my game had changed. I lost the desire to win and with it my smile. This was in the 1970's. This was the same time I began going to work at 3:00 to 5:00 in the morning. My subconscious mind was telling me that I could no longer do complex work in the afternoon. My research involved complex tax research and involved many hours of reviewing tax court cases and the complex tax code as well.

I tried taking a nap after lunch. When I awoke my mind was not able to cope with difficult problems. In the office, I was still out to lunch. I quit working afternoons. I did not know why, but my brain did not function in the afternoon. This was in the 1970's also.

The thought occurred to me that I had suffered a stroke. The plastic look to my face was on the right side; I had a crease wrinkle from the right corner of my mouth to my chin. I started to drool from that side. I was afraid to ask.

I faked it and fooled myself. I did not work in the afternoons, but worked seven days a week. This was during the filing season only, January through April 15th each year. I was semi-retired.

My right leg would tire and cramp. I lost my balance and would stumble at times, as if I were drunk. In the late 1980's these clues became more apparent — impossible to ignore. I was distressed and blue.

Other clues appeared from time to time. It became increasing more difficult to talk on the phone. My voice cracked and I had difficulty speaking. When asked simple questions, such as what is my phone number, my mind would go blank. It happened under stress more frequently. My face would turn red and I would perspire when questioned. My hands would go cold at times.

My handwriting started to change. I could not print an "E" with three legs. My printing was smaller. My hand would tire. When tired, I would not read my writing. Clients ask me, "How I could read my notes?"

It was all centered on the right side. Stroke you might think. I drank more and thought it would take away the tremor. It helped in that people thought me drunk rather than mentally deficient. This suffering went on for over ten years.

I was shocked when the Neurologist told me it was Parkinson's. At least it had a name. I was very concerned still and my wife was concerned. We are both concerned today, too.

Dr. DeLong of Emory University has restored hope, if not for a cure, at least for a few good years. I smile again and feel that I have more to give to life. I am now writing.

I suffered for ten years not knowing. I suffered ten years after finding out. I have hope restored and pray the next ten years will be productive. May I have many more reasons to smile!

August 22, 1998
You want to change your job?
September 20, 1998

C. Cameron Piatt, CPA, MBA, CLU, CMA, CFP
119 North Vine Street
Westerville, Ohio 43081

Dear Cameron:

You certainly make me scratch my head in wonder sometimes. If I was half as intelligent as you seem to think, I would be more outspoken and free with my advice.

I don't know what you need to do, but I do know that you need to be challenged. I will regress a few thoughts. You are not me, but you are a seeker. You are at a crossroad; plan your next move, search your soul, be sure, not swift.

The world has changed in the last fifty years. It will change more in the next thirty years. Momism and apple pie are no longer valid concepts. Company loyalties are dead. This is, especially true of mid and higher management jobs.

I call it the baseball and football common sense rule. You can't fire the team, but you can fire the coach and his staff. Get out of private enterprise or have a contract with high penalties for termination.

Demand a stock option or equivalent cash incentive, if the company does well. Leave the amount open ended (ten percent of all profit).

Your retirement and your medical insurance must be negotiated up front. You must have disability coverage.

We have the Ike concept:

1. Big companies don't like termination pay
2. Big companies are self serving
3. They are super political
4. Promises mean nothing
5. Middle size companies use you until you become too expensive, then they bring in a family member.
6. Employment is based upon need of the company, not on the need of the employee.
7. Big companies and little are self seeking

The pot of gold will still be available forever. The carrot is still dangling at the end of the stick. Big companies know that the exotic executive will never accept their demise. The number of executives who cash in on these will be a small percent of yesterday's number.

The lost adage happiness will be rediscovered. It is important to me and should be to you. Seek security. Wealth should be accumulated, by controlled spending. Live within your means; drive a small car until it dies.

You ask what I would do this day, September 19, 1998. You should not go into accounting. The CPA small businessman is underpaid and overworked. His responsibilities are too great, the pressure extensive, the rewards evasive. The CPA profession, as it is this day, is doomed. Computers and data transmission will make home base competition the major player. Fees will be lower, and the pressure will be the same. Partners in the big firms feel they are losing the battle for survival. Don't consider public accounting!

To a less intellectual man, I would suggest a government job. The government protects the employee with disability, retirement, medical, and doesn't work them too hard. The job is almost for life. They seldom fire anyone.

The competition must be analyzed in any job you seek. In government, you will not be competing with many (less than 1%) equal to you in talent and skill. In public accounting, you compete against CPAs.

CPAs have the highest IQs of all the professions. What should you do? I have never been so sure of a position as I am now.

You should be a college professor!

Education is and always has been a prestigious profession. It now pays better than ever before.

Professors earn $75,000 to $120,000 per year. Thirty years from now, they will earn twice that. With their benefit package, they earn far more than public accountants.

With your personality and super credentials, you could be a college president. A secure future is available in education. Your work hours are limited and free time available. Vacations are the best available to a working person.

Go to the most prestigious colleges in your area. Apply for acceptance in their PHD program. Ask for a position as assistant professor. Do it.

Love,
Dad

In the last few years of our marriage, the days were more often like the following.

BOO HOO BOO HOO TUESDAY

Today started off to be a nice one
The sun was due to shine; the dogs were having fun

Sarah's back hurt; the house was trashed
She was mad at the world and low on cash

She attacked Ike with words; a plenty bad scene
Four letter words that were very obscene

The four pups have been poking and peeing
If Ike had a place to go, he would be fleeing

Ike does not know how to pick up shit
He tries, but Sarah yells and throws a fit

Because Ike picks up dog shit, she is mad
Ike cannot even wipe up pee, it is sad

He leaves spots on the carpet when he tries
Sarah is mad at the four pups; Ike's problem, she lies

Sarah has raised hell three times seven
Ike feels so low; it seems like seven times eleven

He does nothing right and is sad to see
Sarah is trying to make him so low, he will no longer be

A man is something he was a long time ago
He is down the sewer river, deep in the flow

It makes Sarah feel superior to put him down
She thinks it is funny; likes to see him frown

The sun shines behind the black clouds above
With a smile on her face, she says, “Its’ love”

Ike says that it smells a lot like poop
He tries to please and jumps through the hoop

He truly wishes she were happy
But she would rather be so snappy

November 24, 1998

VADE LONG IS DEAD

March 14, 1999, at the age of sixty-five, and too young to go
He was a close friend for the last fifty-one years, I know

His goals, were never clear to me, in some ways, he was a stranger.
We spent our youth together, high school, college and the Army, too.

I pulled out some old photographs showing our trip to Mexico in 1955
We had just completed two years of service in the United States Army.

The first post for us was Fort Ord, California, on the ocean above Monterey
We had 16 weeks of basic training and eight weeks of advanced infantry training

The training was over just before Christmas of 1953
We were home for Christmas and I left new years for Germany

Vade stayed on to attend a spy school for a few weeks at Fort Ord
He never would tell me what the school was for, but I deduced that he was some form of security

I was assigned to the personnel department and had access to all the soldiers private records
We assigned the incoming troops to companies as we needed and a few had security clearances

Vade had the security clearance too and these people were assigned to companies
By division orders and not left to our discretion, so we knew they were special

The high point of Vade's service in Germany was when he broke his ankle in a soccer game.
He slept for two weeks straight and was told by the hospital doctors to get off his butt.

We took a week's leave and traveled from Frankfurt to Berlin by rail
Vade and I took in the sights and had a good time, drank a few beers.

I planned to take another trip with Vade and two other buddies in my outfit.
My application for a early release to go to college was approved and I left three months before Vade.

The planned trip to England, Scotland and Ireland, Vade took with my buddies
They had a very good time and George fell in love with an Irish lassie, he later married.

We were able to spend a number of weekends together in Germany
Vade was stationed in Büdingen, about ten miles from my company in Gelnhausen

In college, Vade and I represented the Alpha Tau Omega fraternity in sports,
We played basketball, football, swam and were first team in all.

Vade was on the college swim team, ran the 440, threw the shot put in track, and was a diver as well.

I played tennis, badminton, threw horse shoes, and made it to the quarter finals in the ping pong tournament.

We were both in the top ten for intramural's for ASU in 1956 and 1957.
We loved all sports, went to most of the college games and missed very few in high school.

Vade loved to fish, we spent many weekends on the Colorado River above Yuma, camping out.
He would stay up all night fishing if the catfish were biting.

He never was much of a student; he did not apply himself ever, well hardly ever.
The last semester of college he needed a "B" average to graduate and he did it.

Vade, like I was in high school, was satisfied to pass and did not strive for "A"s.
We had too much fun to worry and there were very few things we did not enjoy.

Herb was our best friend in high school, he was a fisherman, hunter, and always had a steady girl.
Ike talked to one of Herb's sons and was told they buried Herb two days ago.

We often called Herb, when we were together to say hello.
Herb had a breakdown when he was in the army and was in the Veteran's Hospital in Phoenix.

The fishermen three we used to be
The fisherman is now one.

In honor of Vade's passing, I wish to include some unpublished works of his long-deceased mother, Katherine Long.

DREAMS

Weaving a mesh
For poignant dreams
As elusive as a butterfly;
With thought
Trying to catch eternity
In a net

RHYMING

It’s easy to rhyme “Spring with Sing”.
The rhyming “Summer” is a bummer
It’s a ludicrous thing
To rhyme:
“The rooster goosed her”

WRITE I MUST

Write I must.
The urge is great and I don't know why?
Something within calls
And I must answer.
My heart groans from the kind of hurt this is not pain
But an intense joy.
How foolish it sounds when I put it on paper.

It is an excruciating yearning
For my greater self
The self beyond the circle
Of birth and circumstance;
The pregnant void
Of reality
If I labor
I can give birth to the real me,
The boundless expansion of self
To merge with the throbbing rhythm
Of all selfhood
Encompassed in one great pulse of being.

Like an unhatched chick
I peck at my shell.
I hear music and murmurs
And I thrill to the promise

Of freedom and joy on the other side.
In the silent places of my knowing
With complete assurance
I wait for the hour of my release.
In the meantime, I peck away
With persistent prayers
And a longing
That will someday break my shell.

POEM FOR MY SECOND HUSBAND

One day you came along
Singing the same old wondrous song;
How was my heart to know
From the start, I would love you so?

Why is my vocabulary so archaic
When my thinking is not?

I'm getting weary, Lord,
I'm bending beneath my load,
And Robert is getting impatient
To get his show on the road

Senile capers:
In the morning about five
He (surrepticously) touches my arm
—-Not to press his charm—-
But to know, if I'm alive.

THIS IS NOT GOODBYE

This is not goodbye, though life has spent its bloom
And love will never die, the cloth must leave the loom.
Always this was meant to happen; so adieu.
Destiny has sent us, planned this rendezvous.

All of us will meet again to reap and sow
Bitter crops or sweet — the food by which we grow.
Not with heavy steps nor sadness will I roam;
Swift and sure and glad, I turn my steps back home.

This is not goodbye; we'll meet another day,
And like the stars on high, Love will light the way.

MY PRAYER

Oh God, Who gave me children,
Help me to know the way;
Oh guide my heart with counsel;
Teach me to lead, I pray,
The way to climb the mountain,
Guiding with hope and love,
Through barren slopes or flowers;
Looking beyond, above
.Oh let me send them forward
Whether in work or play,
Equipped with faith and laughter;
Daring to go your way.

SECRET LOVE

My heart leaps forward
As he walks along
The shaded walk;
With head held high
And sensitive step,
He passes by.
And he will never know
That my love
Follows him
Down the street;
And that in empty moments
The thought of him
Brings gratitude,
Humility,
A surge of love,
And joy in all I see
Wherever he goes
My love will
Follow him;
—The Blind Boy
With The Dog.

UNTITLED

Where are the chicks
Of twenty-six?

Where are the guys
Who "gave them the eyes"?

Life is not grim
Tho lacking in vim;

And seeing needs light,
And hearing is slight.

And meat they chew well,
If pounded like hell!

To watch an old movie
To them is still groovy.

While she's making booties
For grandbaby cuties,

He waters for hours
The lawn and the flowers.

His pulse doesn't flip
With each shapely hip,

And that nude centerfold
May leave him just cold.

It may come as a sting
To not feel a thing;

But lacking this bliss
He can still reminisce;

Tho approaching December
He still can remember.

And who really can know
That a roof thatched with snow

- Belying the smirks, -
Has a furnace that works!

ME

I am unique, as unique as can be
And no other creature can ever be me.
Mystery of being: a part of the whole
Sharing ubiquitous essence of soul,
Nurtured, sustained by the blood of the Tree;
Fruition reflecting the conscious degree.

Merit is not whether thistle or rose —
The pattern of seed determines what grows.
Roses may wither or fail to fulfill
The hope of the reaper, the dream of the hill,
But rose it will be whether withered or blown,
Delusion or crown to the seed that was sown.

I am the sower, yet I am the root
And I am the reaper gathering the fruit.
God is the substance of Life in the earth,
The Source ever-present, from moment of birth.
Just as the measure I draw in each limb,
That measure's the part of which I am Him.
I, as a being, am whole and complete;
I choose my success; attract my defeat.
Whatever the crystallized pattern at birth,
The food of my thought determines my worth.
I as a being, can never be you —

Each flower of life to itself must be true.
But this I can govern: the beauty I yield.
And that which I am, reflects in the field.

PRETTY GIRL

A pretty girl with a spark of joy
She is a beautiful pearl, a little coy

Be sure she is a lady
All too thin, petite, beautiful baby

The Doctor orders, gain weight
Candy and pastries is her fate

Eat, "We won't let you get fat!"
I will buy you a beautiful, stylish Easter hat

One hundred ten to one hundred twenty pounds should be all right
A Twiggy with curves lost in the night

Found beautiful to behold, and heaven to touch
Easy to fall in love with, it would not take much

MORE REFLECTIONS ON MY LIFE WITH PARKINSON'S

50TH REUNION - GROWING UP

It was a time as I remember, when we were very young
The memory is weak and the song I seek is no longer sung

How can it be so?
How were the well-laid plans changed? I want to know

We sought success in the form of great sums of money the most
Sacrifices we were not interested in, we loved to boast

We had this and that; we had been there and done everything wrong
The truth is we were obscene and didn't hear the song

Children were a high priority on the plan as I remember it to be
Our son does heavy drugs and our daughter is in jail yearning to be free

I hope they will for a long time keep her under lock and key
The only time in thirty years, I don't have to worry about her safety

We have the very best Psychiatrist in the United States
We live in a posh neighborhood, security and guarded gates

We were robbed twice last year and sleep in fear
The house and location were number three on the plan so clear

Number five was to have a close and loving family
The children think they are being cheated, out of their inheritance, by us not dying; apparently

Could it be that the plan was for failure?
Six called for foreign travel, first class and a time to treasure

No time for travel in the past twenty years
The children need us; my wife has not shed a tear

Tomorrow I will be sixty-six and my wife is sixty-five
She plays golf, bridge and has her psychiatrist to survive

She worked the year we were married and washed the dishes twice
Number seven on the plan she changed to read a maid would be nice

I can but wonder what would have happened, if I had not stayed
Number seven was changed not to get the maid, but so she would have it made

Such a lofty plan should be correct in at least one point
The country club we joined had pompous people in a plus joint

We sought a long life, good health; this was number nine on the plan
Both overweight, the wife has sugar diabetes; I have been cut and sewed every way they can

Low on the list was happiness
As we grow old, turn gray; we must admit our plan was a mess

Our priorities were out of order and quite stupid and small
We were seeking the wrong things from the start and headed for a fall

We did attend the reunion and according to plan, with a new car and costly clothes
A leopard does not change his spots; we planned to put on the show of shows

The first friend we met was a retired fireman and his wife a retired teacher
They both wore a smile; their four children were a doctor, a nurse, a teacher and a preacher

They did without took out a loan or two, to send their children to college without frills
The loans are paid; they are in good health, happy, and ready for retirement thrills

We went shopping for plain clothes; thankful we were in old traveling clothes
We changed that weekend, didn't put on a show, did not mention money or woes

Back home we fired our psychiatrist, sold our home, got our daughter out of jail and put our son in a treatment facility
We dropped out of the country club, sold my business and bought a small home out of the city

The past two years we have traveled, not first class, but had a good time
The children are on their-own and doing swell; the two grandchildren are fine

S

eptember 20, 2000
To my Sons and Friends:

What is the greatest fear of this Parkinson's patient? It is not the palsy. The dark and gloomy cloud that carries the threat of the partial or total demented curse, that maybe part of the disease, is my greatest fear.
The shaky hand may still write, but the demented mind can be a shallow mind with nothing worth-while to record.
How does one prove to himself or to his family that he is not demented? I find the river deep, but cannot find the answer I seek.
The lack of the ability to speak in a clear and distinct manner is a black and ugly part of my curse. The telephone has turned into a tyrant; panic leaves me unable to find the words I seek and my voice clouds.
The curse has been visible to me for over ten years and they have been good years. It was my unknown companion for years before and I have few complaints.
The sun still shines behind the dark clouds and the days each one in turn show hope. Hope both for this day and for the tomorrows.
My life is good now and may be better tomorrow. Hope lives within me and I care. I care about you, each one and all, too.
As long as I search for the answer to my greatest fear, it is not here.

Clyde C. Piatt

GOOD-BYE MY FRIEND

A friend of many years is gone; life to soon ends
He was a kind, quiet man who had many friends

The past two weeks I have vainly sought relief
Unable to express my diabolical, painful grief

He was a pleasure to know, had the ability to care
Ever proud of his wife and family, his full life he was happy to share

Never too proud, never arrogant in life's dealings
He was able to express his heartfelt feelings

Our first meeting was almost forty years ago
Content with life's ups and downs, he accepted life with a smile, as we all know

Rick was innocent, but in no way naïve
Slow to anger and difficult to deceive

A fork in the road, he always traveled the happy road
Rick looked at the sunny side of life, no matter how heavy his load

A careful, generous man who did not waste time or money
Paid his way, remembered the days he was short of milk and honey

He never complained about his extensive accounting fees
Rick always said, "Bill me please".

The kind man who shared his time and energy with zest
Delivering meals to the hungry, caring for the needy, he gave his best

We had many breakfast meetings over the years
We discussed life, our joys and fears

Both raised during the great depression
Shared the same lesson

Turn the light off; don't flush if it's yellow
Our parents said, "We are not made of money fellow"

If you don't have anything nice to say, don't say anything at all
The last three years Parkinson's slowed my thinking and movement to a crawl

Rick knew I was in trouble, but not the deep terrors
Rick and Don invited my sons and I to a Lakers basketball game
We picked Don and Abernathy up in LA, then to the game, a happy sharing of Don's fame

Barbara and Rick visited the Grand Canyon last year
We met them in Williams, Arizona — no tears

The food was excellent, the visit the same, rainbow and sunshine
It was a very special, enjoyable time; we shared two bottles of fine wine

Strange things flash before you when a good friend has gone away
Big problems you don't remember, little things rule the day

Rick told me about the trip to Alaska, he liked Denali Park the best
He did not like doing without his Big Mac's, a character test

He always ordered his eggs fried, if I remember right
Ate the whites first and the entire yolk in one bite

Rick retired early and had some great years, life he tasted
He enjoyed his extra time, delivering meals, working out, extra time with the family, the great games Don played; time was not wasted

That evening in Williams, like our almost forty years of friendship, past all too swiftly by
Like the wine and gracious dinner, were a celebration of it all, not a time to cry

As I think of it now, it was a grand way to say goodbye
In all ways, Rick was a big man and a gentleman, now I can cry.

Cameron called from Ohio to say Rick had died, he read it on the Internet
Cameron said, "The Lakers game was a super highlight of his growing up." He was upset

Grown men don't cry, if they feel they do
He was choking and so may you

August 14, 2001

RECKONING

In the beginning, the phone ringing awoke me from a dream
In reality, the dream was not over or so it would seem

In a voice, deep and clear, a man of apparent confidence was looking for his father
His forty-year search was over, he need look no further

The shock was great and the sword apparently two sided
The cut was deep, hurt on one side and guilt on the other abided

The younger man was intelligent, polished and apparently at ease
Somewhat in command of my senses, the forest separated from the trees

The dream part was over and reality was upon us
We settled on common ground and only facts did we discuss

He was concerned with my feeling and did not want to create distress
We did not cross sabers, nor was a work offered under duress

The families were discussed, he was married and had children — two
My wife talked with him briefly and in name I introduced his two brothers, too

The discussion was at all times friendly; no chastisement was offered or meant
The deep sense of guilt I still carry, but the call brought a measure of relief, God sent

A few weeks went by and the brothers exchanged greetings
A year passed and a few months more before we arranged a face-to face meeting

It was a difficult time for me and undoubtedly for him too
The children and the wives were exceptional, apparently without too much stress or adieu

This tale is no story, true it has a beginning, but I trust no ending today
The past cannot change, our meeting was a treasure for me to store away

I would like to thank his father and mother for the loving care undoubtedly given in pleasure
Their son, wife and grandchildren are undoubtedly one of their great treasures

I pray and trust that there will be future meetings
Nothing was done on my part to deserve their kind greetings

My stepson is a fine, upstanding man, whom I respect and love. Through the total mess, he was fair and square, a musician, linguist, and I trust, my friend.

THE AMAZING MAN

People notice, he is different and mysterious about him; they wonder
A good student, astute, but not an overachiever, not a bungler

The path he chose did not appear to be aggressive; you would find him complex and his thoughts deep
Like the Mississippi River on a calm day, silent, determined, possessed, self motivated, a seeker not weak

Secret thoughts, the goals, the searching — he did alone — no one to share
In this alone, he was to himself unfair

One may think him a grasshopper; who played the fiddle
To one unsure, he had a plan; he was a riddle

Talk with him one hour and you knew he had a plan — do you?
Wonder boy — there were times you had to wonder what he would do

This man was determined, dedicated, talented and brave
Unlike Van Gough, the painter, he will be recognized before the grave

Like Robert Frost, the American poet, he loves his wife, family and his music — first his wife
He is determined to have and to hold all for life

Robert Frost did not pay the bills writing poetry, even after universal fame
This man's music will one day pay the bills and he will have universal acclaim

He is a thinker, wise and somewhat shy
His music will one day make us all smile, laugh and sometimes cry

Today the man, strong and wise, has taken a wife
May their journey be fulfilling, creative and both enjoy a happy life

The road he traveled would terrify many and they would quit
People love his music; piece-by piece the puzzle is starting to fit

He loved music, travel, people and languages, too
A quiet gentleman who speaks many languages — never appeared blue

A complex scholar who has a keen perception of the value of time, the dollar and family
He has played on the streets of North and South America, Europe too: accepting coin or playing for free

Talented, dedicated with a keen perception — we greatly admire his grit
We know he is the captain of his ship

His course was charted many years ago
Captain of his ship, it is now his show

The road he traveled alone, the trips throughout the world and his years of study — quite an education
Together may the road be paved in joy and celebration!

Aim high — do not see out for material wants — be free

You have the knowledge, ability and the all-important tenacity

You have the well-honed tools and a reached before goal
Give the world your music and save your soul

September 22, 2001

DON'T THROW IN THE TOWEL

I have been down in six rounds out of seven
Round eight of twelve and I am not ready for Heaven

So far, I have been shadow boxing — have not thrown the right
For those who feel I should call it a night — I have just began to fight

Sir Parkinson is a degrading and unforgiving foe
Shamefully I tried to get him to take a dive — he refused the dough

My manager wants me toe to toe for the remaining rounds
Fight tough, dirty, fair play is out, so it sounds

Dirty is not my way, but I do so want to win
My foe is mean and rough, does not bluff — fears no sin

My wife in the corner — she fears not
My sons are at ringside — they're the only team I've got

My cup runs over so why the long face
As you breathe — you're still in the race

Your foe has been unmasked — don't be sad
Smiles and laughter are still to be had

Pick up your staff; fight off the blues

Smile and this is a fight you won't lose

Set him up with the left jab, an upper cut; shed a tear but don't cry
Dance on your toes, reach to the sky, your foe is going to die

You are bloodied and bruised, soul weary and sore
Win this fight and you will fight nevermore

WHO AM I?

Dust I may be
Without My Love, I cannot see.

Call me home, My Love,
To your Castle by the Sea.

On The White Cliff's of Santa Barbara
Use your sword and set me free.

Dump my ashes over the White Cliffs into the sea.
Where my lost soul can find rest

Kill the ghost of the "Lady in Red"
Set your spirit free, where joy can find you forever more.

If I am to never gaze on the White Cliff's I will die.
I pray happiness find you, swing your sword, I will not cry.

November 30, 2002

Parkinson's has been my companion for over twenty years; in 2002 my wife kicked me out, gave me two hours to pack. 2003 found me with cancer; four types of cancer were described after they roto- tilled half of my prostate away.

Ike has not demanded anything. He cannot afford a ticket to the opera in Fresno. He would like to go. Sarah knew that I could not be left alone. She has told me she is afraid I would burn the house down. I turned the stove on three years ago in Flagstaff and forgot it. Sarah has left for a dental conference in Nevada. Ike was left alone to take care of the dogs. Sarah had neighbors check on me. Ike takes his medications. Sometimes he does not take Paxil if he is not depressed. The last year of Ike's life has been rotten, the worst ever. He loves Sarah and does not want a divorce.

He does not approve of the lies or actions of the manic depressed actions of Sarah. The psychiatrist says she is Bipolar — in the manic stage, she is a mess.

1. She has struck me, a hard punch that left my shoulder black and blue
2. She has kicked me
3. Tried to push me over the cliff (100 foot drop) at her castle by the sea
4. She asks me why I don't die? Why I don't eat a shotgun? Bang! Calls me gutless and a wimp.
5. She tore up sixty to ninety art pieces, broke vases, etc, threw them at me

The doctor says I have all the symptoms of Parkinson's — Sarah says, I have "a few of the symptoms, when I don't take my medicine."

Sarah has ordered me to go to my room many times because I can't talk or have extensive uncontrolled twitching — arms, legs, hand, and body.

Sarah is abusive and said I was homeless. Jon, my son, ordered me to leave his home; it was hot. Jon gave me a check for $600 and ordered me to pack and leave. He said my three plus carat gold ring would be security. Jon said, "I could not get more from the pawnshop."

I moved into a motel. I was sick, exhausted and broke. The pawnbroker had loaned me $4,000, on my watch. They loaned me $800 more on my sterling silver and my new wedding ring. I still had the car as a last resort. Sarah, without being asked, gave me a car. She picked it out and did ask me if I liked it. It was a beautiful automobile and would fit the image; Sarah said she wanted me to be a country gentleman, a squire, wealthy with fine jewelry and nice clothes.

Sarah said, "I was greedy." I never asked for a car, clothing or money. No Never. I did ask for a caring, loving wife. I loved her and she was told so many times. Sarah told me she would give me, $1,000,000 and, an income after taxes, of $5,000 to$6,000, a month. She gave me $100,000; a lot of money with no strings attached. I gave Sarah a list of expenses and cash outlays that accounted for over $100,000. She ignored that list.

She gave her children ten times the amount she gave me. She has bought them similar amounts of jewelry, etc. I did not and do not object to these gifts. Children should be taken care of and she gave new cars to the grandchildren.

Sarah promised to put her granddaughter's husband through medical school — a gift of $500,000 or more. Sarah's gifts to me were less than ten per cent of those gifts to others. Sarah blows her horn about being so generous to Ike. She kicked Ike out of the house; gave Ike two hours to pack. If he was not out, she would throw him out and trash any goods he left. Sarah, without telling me about it, had secretly met with Chip, her attorney, the day before on October 10. The week before, she had told her children that she "LOVED IKE" and DID NOT want him to leave.

Shawn, Marsha, and Celeste had told Ike that "They Loved Him", but thought he should leave for a while. Ike thinks that, they were afraid Sarah would kill Ike, in one of her Manic Stages. Greed is part of the problem. Sarah's problem: She was open and generous before. She repeatedly told Ike, "He would not get a penny for support from her." She never gave me the monthly expense account promised.

Not one penny was given to Ike during 2002 or 2003, until the court ordered it.

Ike's assisted living costs are $83.00 per day (31 x $83 = $2,573 a month). It has forced me from a comfortable lifestyle to a borderline poor lifestyle. Drinking is a non-existing problem. I do not drink. Maybe a glass of beer with Mexican food, or a half a glass of wine once a month, is not drinking. Sarah has told my family, friends, and neighbors that I am not capable of taking care of myself.

I could not drive, but limited mornings, etc. Sarah attests to my being able. It would appear that I have been cured. I can work, etc. Sarah states that I lied about the standard of living.

Sarah insults my intelligence when she swears under oath that I indicated that "I was selling my securities and using the money to gamble. Such a big lie! It may be believed by an ultra demented person. It was very insulting and demeaning to me.

I do not gamble my savings, only a small amount of dollars for entertainment. You cannot win and I don't like paying for Vegas' light bills.

My all time high loss was in Las Vegas in 1978. My wife and I were guests at the Sands for a week. I stayed three days in a golf tournament with a group of businessmen from San Francisco, Los Angeles, and Santa Barbara. We were asked to bring no money as they "The Casino" paid for everything. We were given a line of credit in the casino and hotel. Harris Seed and Robert Montgomery were among the guests from Santa Barbara. I paid $900, when, I checked out. Our golf, luxury meals, rooms, and shows were compensated. We received $2,000, plus for golf, shows, meals, etc.

My trips to Reno, Tahoe, Las Vegas, over the past eighteen years, probably averaged three to four per year. Sarah was there. The most I ever lost in a trip was $350.00.

This letter was written to my third attorney in Santa Barbara, California.

December 4, 2003

Paul Roberts
200 East Carrillo Street Suite 310
Santa Barbara, California 93101
Tel: 805-963-7400
Fax: 805-963-7610

Tammy:

1. Please mail me a copy of the November 13 and 14, court trial.
2. Send me a recap of the requested and the court approval regarding legal fees.
3. Did the court set a date for payment?
4. Do I have any rights re: approval of the agreement? Do I have the right to make one or two five-minute calls a week?
5. Do I have the right to demand access to the notes re: negotiations as they proceed on a day to day basis, on a weekly basis? Or is it required that I wait until completion?
6. Demand is and always has been a last resort to me, but I have dealt with over fifty attorneys in Santa Barbara and have never been treated so without respect.
7. I have great difficulty in phone conferences and writing, but most of the time, I am acutely aware of the place, time, goals and the reasons for my involvement. My thinking ability, even slowed by age and medical problems is confidentially higher than average.
8. My ability to recognize truth has never been sharper.
9. Your acceptance of my position is not important to me personally___
10. But probably affected your lack of interest and lack of conviction re: my life style standard of living during marriage.
11. Other than the unfortunate word choices of Diane, I attempted "TO TELL THE TRUTH!" She did not give me the time to meet

with her either. I signed the filed papers. Things like: "Jet plane, two engine prop Cessna" should have been corrected.

12. The lies told by Sarah, Marsha, Sandra, my Son, Jon, Gae and Lisa, my daughter-in-law, HURT. They were bad.

13. The personal slander stressing DRINKING and GAMBLING PROBLEMS were painful. THEY WERE LIES!

14. The Judge was concerned; by the denied and contested statements, by me. He accepted the lies. He accepted the statements by Sarah and Skip to be true.

15. If Sarah is not paying ASAP, I have to borrow my rent monies.

a. I have received a final bill from Paul.

b. Does he still represent me?

c. Do I call the Judges' office regarding monies due me, and the life insurance question?

d. Today is December 4, and no payment has been received!

e. Clyde C. Piatt

The past three years have been filled with terror, and at times death stalked me. The grim reaper was after me and was on my mind every hour. He visited me every night, left me wet with perspiration and shaking from fear.

My wife's mother died in April 2002. She had an estate in excess of one hundred million dollars. My wife and her brother inherited the estate along with the family charitable foundation. My wife and I moved into the family estate house in Santa Barbara, California in April 2002. She often told me she loved me. We still held hands.

She went on a spending spree and managed to spend: Jewelry - $440,000; Cars - $240,000; Home Improvements - $1,300,000; Gifts to Children - $1,000,000;One time tax free transfer for her Mother's estate.

I was her Mother's CPA. Sarah's children approached me. "They were concerned their mother was losing control and would spend all the money." I thought she was blowing a few dollars, but could not spend enough to hurt her financially.

Martha, her mother had given Sarah very little over the years. Martha, when asked to help Marsha, who was sick, with a neurological problem; she said, "No!" Marsha had seen all the specialists in Santa Barbara and Sarah thought John Hopkins Hospital in Washington might help. Martha had given John Hopkins a few million dollars in donations, over the years. She was a board member of John Hopkins. Martha told Sarah that John Hopkins was expensive. She offered no assistance and no support.

I was sure that having a rich parent who gave you very little; it was nothing in light of the funds her Mother had available. She still had me doing her accounting and I assured her children, their estate was safe.

My wife rebuilt the home and installed a Jacuzzi for me. The massager and heat were a blessing for the Parkinson's. We went out for dinner every night and lived the life rich people live. She bought gifts for everyone: Car for Sarah — Jaguar, $48,000; Car for me — BMW Z-3 Touring Coupe, $44,000; Watch for me — Rolex, $20,000; Watch for me — Rolex, $10,000; New Wedding Rings — Diamond & Gold, $5,800; Clothing (one shopping day), $3,500; Cash — check to me, $50,000; Cash — check to me, $50,000. Total for the period May 1, 2002 through October 14, 2002: $231,300.

Sarah gave me a diamond and gold watch and a gold watch. These watches had matching ones for Sarah. She kicked me out on October 12, 2002. I found out later, she had a secret appointment with an attorney the day before she kicked me out. He was her divorce attorney.

The kids, that I had helped raise, told me the week before that they loved me, asked me to leave to see if this separation would help Sarah. Sarah told them, at the time, "She did not want me to leave; she loved me."

The attorney told Sarah that she would have to pay me support and the longer I stayed in the ocean front home, the more support she would have to pay. The poor sick ex-spouse is entitled to maintain their standard of living. The house and four lots were valued at fifteen to thirty million dollars. Money versus love and money wins every time.

I told my wife I loved her and did not want to go! She gave me two hours to pack and leave. Any goods left would be thrown away.

Sarah had a mental breakdown the previous month. She was not in her right mind. The

Psychiatrist had told the family she was suffering from MD — Manic Depression. She was manic.

The girl I loved and married seventeen years before was gone. Money took her away.

I should not have been driving. I was distraught and ill in my fifteenth year of suffering from Parkinson's. I drove seventy miles to Santa Maria, where I spent the night with a cousin.

The next day, I drove to Fresno and moved in with my son, Jon Piatt. It was agreed that I would stay a maximum of six months, with Jon. I planned to spend the next six months with my son Cameron, in Ohio.

The divorce dragged on and I could not leave Fresno where my attorney lived. I had $60,000 cash when we separated. It was going fast, over $30,000 in a six-month period. My car was bought for cash and I had no payments and no credit card debt.

When Jon evicted me, he gave me one day to move. Cameron flew to Fresno from Ohio the next day and we moved my personal goods. Jon and I did not have a fight and I was not aware of any problems between us. I love Jon and God knew I had always liked, welcomed Lisa and respected her opinions. God says to love your neighbor. I love Lisa and wish her well. I believe I am a well-mannered gentleman. I bathe daily, dress well, pay for myself, and help when I can.

I gave Jon and Lisa an $11,000 gift, a few months before my operation. I put Jon through college and he lived in style for twenty years.

Jon did not lift a finger to move me out. It was a hot day in Fresno, 106 degrees. Jon had two trucks. He refused to let Cameron borrow the old truck to move me. Cam and I rented a van. I was sick, had a hernia tear and a prostrate problem. Cam was hot and working under pressure.

My problems were increasing daily. Cameron moved me to an assisted living home. Cam had to return to Ohio and I had an appointment with the VA Hospital in San Francisco for a deep brain operation.

Cam would fly to San Francisco for the operation. Hank Redondo and Don Thompson, from San Diego, would pick me up in Fresno and drive me to San Francisco in a Motor Home.

ROUND TWO - PARKINSON'S IS DOWN

Up in the morning early, feeling bright and thinking clearly
Breakfast, the morning paper and nothing to fear

The beeper rings, it is 7:00, time for the days first pills
At 10:30, it is pill time again, no time to cheer

The mind is starting to slow down
I walk and I talk more like a clown

The shake has gone for a time it is true
It is the fog that, in truth, makes me feel blue

The doctors at Emory said the pills were to blame
Cut back on the pills, shake a little, but feel sane

The blues are not as certain, but come on occasion still
Life is much better and I have climbed another hill

More hills are on the horizon I know, bring them on, I am ready
The body shakes, but the mind is clearly steady

God is my Master and Captain of my ship until I die
My head is bloodied, but my spirit is unbowed and spry

THE SAINTS BE WITH YOU

As they were with me
Three trips to the emergency

These trips to the hospitals
Fresno VA Hospital, San Francisco & St. Agnes

The pain pills took me on a trip
I wandered the halls, alone and sick

An angel took me by the hand
She was sent by the Man

I feared death was stalking me
The Resident Priest absolved me of past sins

Gave comfort to this lost soul
Walked with me without dole

Two weeks she nursed me
My mind cleared and I awoke

I feared my mind had left
I had no memory and was adrift

The angel's loving touch; St. Agnes' angel nurse I love
She saved my life with help from above

The nights were few, when I was sane
I loved this angel; cannot put out the flame

It was a month ago; I left
The angel is in my prayers daily

A voice tells me she must stay
St. Agnes has other patients who need an angel

The angel's name is Heather
The "Golden Years" I need someone who can see

God, please lend her to me
Heather is real and is free

I would like to see the United States once more
A slow trip, a vacation, I cook and sew

To the roads end
A Happiness Treat

St. Agnes please lend her to me
While I am still able and also free

My ex-wife called, the former Las Vegas dancer
Told me she "wished I had brain cancer"

Not a walk in the park with your lover
Twenty years and the fight is not over

HEATHER

In Rome fifty years ago, was my last confession
He gave me absolution

Would my God be so forgiving
Why fight? Was my life worth living

Divorced by my love after twenty years
Fighting an eighteen year battle with Parkinson's

My eldest son perjured himself
He told the court I was no good

A Rolex watch for his wife and one for him
Paid to my son as pieces of silver in years gone by

He chose a stepmother rich and mean
To a Father who loves him sick and poor

Parkinson's, divorced, broken-hearted, homeless and alone
He is angry with me.

I wish I were a righteous man
I am not

Job is a frightful story to me.
One week after meeting the angel Heather

I was told I had prostate cancer
Suicide is not the answer

Heather has given me hope
I am too old to elope

Young enough to be a loving friend
Until the time my story ends

I toured the whole United States in 1976
I would like to show it to Heather

A FRIEND

Depressed, tired, sick, my sun had lost its shine
It does not require a long time

Love at first sight happens rarely
Life does not treat everyone fairly

You and Cloud brightened days and months cast out for me
I was lost, blinded, distraught, free?

You shared your life
A friend you will always be

I could not say goodbye
Big men don't cry

We will meet one day at Gray Eagle
Break bread, play golf, smile and giggle

A beer for Cloud, a golden rainbow for Marie
The golden years past, debts paid and pain free

He will take us in
Sin forgiven friends united again

I was lost, sick, ill, and bewildered
You were cast in with me

I had lost my smile
Your kind words and care

Eased my hurt and time slipped by
You shared your life, listened to my mournful cry

The smile has returned

RISE AND STAND FOR THE BLACK MAN

He's graduated from high school
He graduates from college
Or he's a graduate of the streets
Surviving off of street knowledge
He's gone from being a man to a child
To a rebellious wild child
To a child that you could never understand
Now he's hounded with problems
Too much for the man
Don't tell people such stuff as this
You cannot understand
His future was determined before his birth - Bull
If only you've known all that he's been through — I may be He
He's been beaten, tried and put on a cross to sacrifice — True
He's been enslaved, hung and has risked his life — True
He has marched, demonstrated, and reveled his dream — Not all
He's been jailed, converted to Muslim, and fought for freedom — Not all
By all means (necessary) — Threat
He's being pulled from his family to fight a confusing battle
Hint: for another man, a theft, a liar with President for a title — Not True
He's not perfect. He is just a man.

And when he's fallen short the victory, he needs you to stand. — A person who cannot understand? Why?
Society has broken the pride that resides in his chest.
He was born with expectations for failure — Not by Me
Never to do his best — Bull
"They" didn't want him to rise tall enough to stand — A Lie
He was never expected to live long enough to reach the age of man — A Lie
Very few can see the beauty within him — Good
Because the light that used to shine,
Is now lowered and dim
You can see the pride if you look deep into his eyes,
When he speaks you'll hear that his educated, determined and wise.
He has a love so deep if you stand by him long enough to realize,
That when a black man falls, he needs you to rise
Stand for the man who is trying — I Do
Stand for the black man whose soul is dying — I Do and include all rain, lo colors, not only Black
Stand for the man in the times and do rags,
Even the ones who prefer for their pants to sag.
Stand for the actor who won our first Oscar — Yes
Stand high the black men who have become our doctors — Yes
Stand for the little man who's standing for his daddy — O.K.
Even if he's stunting as a candy-painted Caddy — O.K.
Stand for Barack Obama with dreams for a change
Stand for the man who's surviving, begging for pocket change — No Need
Stand for the man who has planted our seeds — Tend the crop, harvest and see from beginning to end
Don't plant the seed and run away.
Stand tall for the man who caters to a woman's needs — The family needs a father
For through God I was produced from the rib of a black man
Because I am he and we are one
I will forever rise and stand

BLACK AND WHITE

The local newspaper is one of gloom and doom
Its main subjects are bombs, murder and death, too soon

Do people really buy it because of the stories?
We all have more than we need of worries

There are many stories worth the telling
Still they print stories, like Nazi crowd's yelling

We have the police who watch these few member groups
It is worthwhile news when the governor calls out the troops

Anything less is not worth the bother, to my brother
It is a pure waste of time and insulting to my mother

There are a few good newspapers without local news
Many can't afford two newspapers, we must choose

It would please me to see a separate section, for trash
Include the murder, rapes and robberies, and cars that crash

Tell us of flowers blooming, their color and their fragrance
Tell us of marriages, medical advances, travel in France

We all know that everything that happens is not good
Print a good newspaper, we want it and you should

TIGER AT 30

Twenty years of suffering from Parkinson's.
I played golf for fifty-one years.
The last round at Gulf Port
That last game, I shot a ninety-six
Drove my drive one hundred-fifty yards
I love the game
I love Tiger Woods
I am with you for every shot
I enjoy Bam-Bam Couples,
John Daly, Gary Player, Nickels, Palmer
My last ten years, you chased away the pain for a few hours.
You are a remarkable man.
You could be the finest president, a professional golfer
The success of your foundation can support and verify your leadership ability.
I would support a man such as you.

1. Intelligent
2. Truthful and Honest
3. A Giver, who shares time and wealth
4. A dedicated and tireless worker

I never lost faith in you.
You never were meant to win all the tournaments,
You honor your Father and Mother
Give God a little press
We must not forget him.

You chase away blues
Give me cause to smile
I pray records will fall.
You remain undaunted by all.

PIATT V. PARKINSON'S, ROUND 19

Parkinson's has been a curse of Job — my "stations of the cross". Peter aided Christ and Jesus Christ has aided me. Without the help, I would not be in my twentieth year of this disease.

It was a short time, a time to smile and a time to cry. I have completed my book,

"PARKINSON'S THE CURE 2007"; the notes, letters and stories are true and I still have hope. I had a doctor's appointment this morning. They will treat the prostate cancer with radioactive isotopes seeds". It is good news. The isotopes are the winners 85% of the time.

I have been to the river, have been baptized, but I am not ready to throw in the towel. The rounds pile up and I somehow answer the bell. It is a championship fight and the rounds are unlimited. I am bloodied, feet are heavy, tired and weary, but I have just begun to fight.

Soon the "thunderbolt" right will strike

Parkinson's will soon vanish with God's might.

Michael J. Fox has a similar history and we fight the same foe. I most admire his tenacity and grit. His work to challenge Parkinson's is without a peer. He is the uncrowned champion. Michael's TV and movie career has survived the shakes. He puts his left hand into his pocket, carries a book, etc, wears a poncho or serape, turns away from the camera and goes on with his acting. His courage and skill have given me many hours of relief, and a few laughs. He should receive an Oscar and not life. The pressure of appearing before Congress results in gross uncontrolled jerks. Michael probably chose to show the world, he was fighting, determined to win the battle against the malignant monster, Parkinson's.

We will someday find a cure. Mohammed Ali has done a great job and is a champion — his public appearances shaky and in pain. He still climbs the stairs and roars his challenge to Parkinson's,

"You can't beat me, I am the champion".

"Float like a butterfly; sting like a bee"

Parkinson's you will soon be down for the count

A mighty right by Mohammed Ali

Mohammed Ali, along with Michael J. Fox, heads a research foundation looking for a cure.

Mahlon R. DeLong, MD, Chairman, Head of Neurology at Emory University is a renowned world leader in the race for an answer. I have been a patient there since 1988. He is the author of many papers about the treatment of Parkinson's. Dr. DeLong's wife is an alchemist and the treatment of Parkinson's in patients requires a mastery of all the available drugs. The combinations are endless and the results vary from patient to patient. The Doctor must be a master detective — STUDY, STUDY, STUDY each case. REVIEW, REVIEW, REVIEW each patient's reaction. He must be flexible. Combinations may work for some, but not all. The medications may work for six months or six years. The detective work is incessant and demanding.

The Doctor must be persistent in his challenge, thorough in his research, a master of diagnostic technique. He must care. He often can give ten years of living to a patient as opposed to ten years of dubious battle. He may work miracles without a permanent cure.

He has released me from bondage of Parkinson's. Gave me hope and returned my ability to smile. The first visit with Dr. DeLong, there were three neurologists who spent 3 ½ hours examining me. Dr. DeLong personally spent 2 ½ hours with me.

I have been under the care of a Neurologist at Sansum Medical Clinic in Santa Barbara,

California, Roseville Neurologist in Sacramento, California, Veterans Administration in Prescott,

Arizona, Mayo Clinic Neurologists in Phoenix, Arizona, Veterans Clinic in Santa Barbara, California, The Brain Institute in Fresno, California, Veterans Administration in San Francisco, California, and the Neurology Department at St. Agnes Hospital in Fresno, California.

I have been examined by twenty-two Neurologists, in the past nineteen years. In most cases, the first examination takes one half hour. This does not include clerical time or testing done by the staff.

The VA Doctor in Columbus, Ohio fills out my monthly prescriptions. He reduced Sinemet from 390 tabs. Carbloopa 25/ Levodopa 100 mg Tabs to 360 Tabs.

He is afraid I am taking a dangerous overdose. I told him, "I wake up every hour and without the Sinemet, I shake uncontrolled and can't get out of bed, cannot walk.

He feels I need to be tough. I have suffered through a big, angry monster, who dispenses pain with joy in his soul, a black angel. This black angel derives pleasure from my pain. This suffering started in 1980 and the pain just gets worse with each passing day. I have suffered over twenty years.

I told the VA Doctor that his examination is routine and he does not experiment with medications. He will not prescribe or recommend anything except Sinemet.

Sarah held up for ten years into the fight with Parkinson's. She began to lose control with reality. She told me she loved me at a family meeting five days before she kicked me out. She had been in the Santa Barbara County Psycho Ward a few weeks earlier. She had a mental breakdown and also suffered from Bells Palsy.

Love turned to hate. She said, "You tricked me in to marrying you." The love notes and cards she gave me tell a different story. I believe she loved me. Parkinson's killed the love. She inherited thirty to sixty million dollars, six months before the divorce. She told me she wanted the money to go to her children. I know that I was the victim of Parkinson's and kicked out by her greed and fear of a claim by me.

Sarah met with a divorce attorney on October 14, 2002, the day before greed and she told me to leave. She gave me two hours to pack all I could into the new BMW roadster she had given to me two months earlier.

She gave me a twenty thousand dollar Rolex Watch, a new wedding ring, a new wardrobe and told me she was giving me a million dollars. She promised a monthly income of five to six thousand dollars, so I could live like a rich gentleman. She gave me two fifty thousand dollars checks too.

The day after, she sneaked off and met with the attorney, she "HATED ME" and gave me the boot. Was it greed? Did the attorney tell her that I may be entitled to support?

Care givers are under a great strain and many divorce their Parkinson's partners. They are capable of murder. Sarah told me, "She hired a hit man to kill me."

I did not announce that I had Parkinson's for six or seven years. The disease is difficult to recognize for the untrained. When I fell, I was thought to be drunk — better a drunk then a demented soul.

Sarah took care of me the first few years. She did not baby me. I had all the responsibility for medications and planning. I drove between Santa Barbara and Lake Wildwood monthly for seven and a half years with Parkinson's. Sarah made most of the trips the first two years. I pushed myself hard, but continued my CPA tax practice for ten years with Parkinson's

She went to work for a dentist in Flagstaff. She bought three new cars the last two years in Flagstaff and lost $20,000 on the cars. This was more then she earned working. She went to work to get away from me and escape Parkinson's.

A letter to my son follows. I want him to know me.
Jon Piatt
Fresno, California

August 16, 2004

Dear Jon:

It is a very strong hurt that is consuming me. I was deeply hurt when you told me you "would knock me on my butt", some twenty one years ago.

You stayed with me and visited me many times over the past twenty years. You cared and it showed. I love you son, and wish you and Lisa the best. You care or you would not have visited me many times. I pray you will come to realize that your brother and I care for you. We are both concerned. You are an important part of the family.

You kicked me out, but the other side of the coin was, I was invited to stay for six months. I over-stayed my invitation by three months.

Sarah is sick and is not the girl I married. I love the girl I married and it would be a blessing to see her return. She is using money for power and the "power" is from hell.

Keep your guard up. She is in her "manic state", is capable of murder. She tried to push me over the cliffs.

You are welcome any time and I will forget the bad times.

Sarah needs help and I pray she gets it. Her father died forty-five minutes after I arrived from Santa Barbara. I held his hand and talked with him for over thirty minutes. I called the nurse and told her, "Sarah's father had suffered enough." The nurse gave Allan a shot and he died two minutes later.

Sarah's father would not appreciate Sarah's new self either. He was a great, kind Jewish gentleman. He waited for me to arrive after April 15, 1992, before he would die. He died in Mobile, Alabama on April 17, 1992.

Son, there is nothing you did, could do or have done that I cannot forgive. I miss you and will suffer until this trial has passed.

I feel like Job must/should have felt. I wish I were a righteous man, but I am a sinner.

Repentant and sorry, though I be. Parkinson's, kicked out and divorced in 2002, prostate operation in March 2004, and a cancer operation in August 2004.

Told to leave by my son; a sick old man of seventy. If not for Cameron, the next place for me was on the street.

Cancer will not defeat me
Soon happy times will greet me
And you will see
The truth will survive
I will live to one hundred and five
The Parkinson's will be cured before I die

Love,

Dad

Dear Marion and Cloud:

The past five months have found me in limbo where I remain.
Telling friends about my troubles seems insane.

You have better things to do with your time.
I owe you an apology

My eyes are open, but I do not see.
The stories and happy meals we shared were therapy.

The stories exchanged and conversation sustained me.
It saved me from dubious battles of self-pity

.
You and Cloud, Betty, Bill, Elizabeth, Mary and the entire staff were there with me.
I could not say "goodbye" … I would cry — not for friends to see.

The sun still shines, but the black, menacing, bleak clouds hides it.
I am getting better day by day — bit by bit.

Next week, August 12, 2004, it is operation time again.
Radioactive seeds will be planted; this battle I will win.

The blues will surely leave me; I will be cancer free.
My son, Cameron will be forty. He has great plans for his son; we shall see.

His wife, Becky is expecting in January, their first, a boy. Hallelujah!
Caleb Cameron Piatt was born November 12, 2004.

He weighed almost five pounds.
The event gives me cause to rejoice.
No happenstance blessing after many years trying — a blessing by choice.

Time to live — no more crying
A God sent sign — no more thoughts of dying.

My leaving was a hegira, a journey, a departure to flee.
An undesirable situation — the correction you gave me is still unclear; sorry.

Three weeks in the hospital was pain and suffering misery.
Ohio is beautiful and I am, at last, pain free.

SUMMER IS GOING SOUTH EARLY THIS YEAR

Summer visited a few days this year.
July, August and September passed by without a cheer

The year 2004 is closing fast.
No spring, no summer followed by a mild winter … it just passed.

Please don't skip the painted leaves of October, beautiful!
Time, we pray, will stop running by; may the judge be dutiful.

We pray the seasons return.
The honking geese last night signaled their return and winter is on their heels.

Winter has been too long, too cold and nasty.
The groundhog saw his shadow; six more weeks of winter, we need tenacity.

Trust our resident groundhog finds a mate.
To live alone is not Plato's fate.

September 9, 2004

THE ROBINS ARE HERE

December 1 in Ohio, the day not cheery, but rather cold, overcast and dreary.
The Robins look like they lost a way, they are weary.
Hungry, tired and in a hurry to leave, Florida bound they must scurry.

They could use a little sunshine,
A good meal, worms are fine.

They must dine and dash, no time for conversation.
Robins only pass through on their migration.

They say hello and in a day or two
The robins are gone. They were just passing through.

No good bye, but we were glad they stopped by.
Like the years, they come and go, we must not cry.

December 1, 2004

Sarah called the hospital six times and acted concerned. I hoped she was over her manic depression. I will learn later that she was not. She called a seventh time to Outlook Manor. She said, "I hope you get cancer of the brain." Her manic depression is back. I pray she gets well.

The days go by slowly. I am still not feeling well. They will operate again on August 12, 2004 to insert radioactive "seeds" of Iodine 125 in the prostrate. This will kill the cancer. They did a good job; the plumbing works and no sign of cancer.

This was done as planned. I still have dog days, six out of seven. The radiation sickness has robbed me of all energy and is still stealing my energies today.

I have a grandson, Caleb Cameron Piatt, born November 12, 2004. God has heard my cries. He is a gift from God and is GREAT. God did a very good job on Caleb. They have no plans for more children, but I am thankful for one. Time to quit crying. Time to get well. I am trying.

December 4, 2002

Dear Sarah:

You have, many times, asked me for a figure. My estimated monthly living costs are as follows. Mortgage Payment: $2,168; Food: $800; Utilities: $400; Medical Expenses: $1,500; Automobile: $600; Travel: $600; Medical Insurance: $280; Entertainment: $460; Misc: $400. This sub-total is $6,148. The taxes on the home are $440 and Income taxes are $3,000. This constitutes a total monthly expense of $9,588 or $115,065 annually.

You provided the following support for 2002: Cash gift of $50,000; Cash gift of $50,000; Wrist watch #1: $10,000; Wrist watch #2: $19,000; Wedding ring: $3,000; Clothing: $3,500; Kangaroo leather hat: $90 for a sub-total of $176,500. You also purchased meals out totaling $4,500; the rental at the Flagstaff property in the amount of $12,000; 7-months shared rental at the Santa Barbara property totaling $35,000 and automobile expenses of $12,000. The total support provided to me was $235,500.

You promised me a million dollars in cash. You said you would provide a monthly income to me, of $5,000 to $6,000 a month. This would have been after tax income. It will be double that amount ($6,000 x 2 = $12,000) if taxable.

I would like to rent from you half of the master bedroom for six months a year at $3,000 per month or $18,000 per year. This would be accomplished by reducing your monthly payment, to me, by $3,000 per month (x 6 months). This would be for your care and rent. The other six months, I will contract Lisa and Jon for care.

I love you and would like you to love me as you have in the past. The years in Alabama were happy years. We have learned much and can respect and love again. You could arrange for me to visit Jon any weeks, by sending me to Jon's.

I love you and your family, too. They hurt me deeply by not ever giving me a call, when they knew I was worried deeply, concerned about your illness.

They love me, but not one called. When Marsha told you "I sounded like the Monsignor", it stunned me. Your mother left the Monsignor a million dollars and gave him the Polo Club condo. He sold it for $500,000.

My dear Sarah, you have a past marriage agreement that would protect your children from any claims against your estate. It can be a part of the Divorce or a financial agreement of a married couple. I don't want a divorce. You have stated before that you did not want a divorce. Change your name, if you must — that will hurt enough.

If I could be with you three months and with Jon three months, you would have free time and will be cared for, by those who love you. You can be free and still love me. Try it; we can divorce later. What is to be will be.

Love,
Clyde Cleveland

The following note was written to my son, Jon and his wife.

Dear Jon & Lisa,

I miss you and wish you happy sailing.
May the wind be always behind you, no time wasted talking.

Predestination may slow our resolve.
But the little problems, we must still solve.

An unlocked gate
No one's fault; it was fate.

The stock gone, the gate locked
The ship is securely docked

True uncharted waters lie ahead.
Face them, I must, I will, I am not dead.

"To everything there is a season, a time for every purpose under Heaven."

Ecclesiastes 3:1
Clyde C. Piatt
December 21, 2004

FOR A GRANDSON

Dear God, Omnipotent One,

I am three. In nine months I will be one.
Life is beautiful and lots of fun.

How do I pray to thee?
Your wonderful world I want to see.

You say, "Your work was good."
Your ability, wonderful and unlimited, it should.

Grandpa praises all Your work.

He wants You to know, You did a very good job on me.
Wonderful and beautiful are your creations of land and sea.

I want to know You and serve You happily.
Your world is great, so much to see.

Lord, I give my love to Mother, Dad and Thee.
Please remember my Grandpa; he, too, loves me.

I love Grandpa too.
Love my neighbors, all creatures, big, little and tiny, I do.

But most of all, God, I love thee
Marvelous world; so much to see

I love you Dad, most of all, I love You, God, for all Eternity.
The Father, the Son, and the Holy Spirit, the Trinity.

Signed by Clyde C. Piatt
January 15, 2005

PARKINSON'S

Parkinson's has robbed me, embarrassed me, and has led me back to prayer. Our Savior has told us, "He will never give us more than we can take."

The thought of suicide drops in for a visit a few times a year. My Savior has given me the strength to dismiss these thoughts.

I have been told by a few would be friends that, "they would not suffer." My wife told me, "If you had any guts, you would be like Shorty." Shorty was a friend of her mother who put a rifle in his mouth. He died three days later in the hospital…a mess.

I still have good days and enjoy life. It is true, I suffer, but on my worst day, I have three or four good hours. Hope sustains me.

There will be a cure; not within the five year period many of us prayed for. I have been sick for nineteen years and have not lost hope. It may be this year, 2005 has a good sound.

January 22, 2005

It has not been easy and I have offended God whom I have loved as long as I remember. My memory is remarkable and often reminds me of items I would like to forget. I have broken down, yelled, screamed and ranted, pleaded for help, felt like Job. Tears of anger, hurt and frustration — sobs big and begging, asking for help.

Tonight I was watching the ballgame when I was told He had a message for me. My Bible was open to page 423. I was told to add 11 pages and to read that page. It was the last page of the story of Judith. The message appears to be clear. I should not seek a wife or girlfriend. I should spend my time helping others — being a good Christian. Judith lived to 105 years of age. Judith's husband died. She never remarried and was without men until she died at 105.

I don't like living alone, but "His message is clear". The church rules are clear, but current policy would probably grant me an annulment. I did not receive communion from 1954 through 2003. It pained me, worried me and I needed it. The last time I received communion was at St. Peters in Rome, in1954. I practiced birth control and finally conceded to my conscience — I could not make a good confession. I still practiced birth control.

LATE NIGHT VISITOR

I had a late night visitor, never seen before.

She was followed by a teacher; Mother Superior in days gone by.

Last seen in 1948, the teacher seemed relaxed and bid me not to worry.

The other visitor, a lady dressed in blue and white, I had never seen before.

She did not speak, but seemed to say "relax, you will survive."

Her beauty not apparently over powering or flamboyant;

It was there none-the-less and love flowed and comforted.

I had prayed to the two for many years.

They were first introduced to me in 1944.

The teacher, Mother Superior of the Immaculate Conception School in Yuma, Arizona, was Sister Justine.

They had looked after me when I was lost and searching.

They gave me a blue and white flag to care for, display and proclaim my love for "Christ the King."

The teacher had recommended me as a leader (to the high school principal).

Four years of high school, I tarried, played and cared not.

Years later the principal told my father "Sister Justine (Mother Superior) had never been wrong before".

Guilt plagued me evermore.

Was their late night visit a "we forgive you"?

Maybe it was an announcement. "Now is the time to even the score."

Make amends; we will help as in all the years gone by.
You are not alone, do not cry."
A DREAM OR WAS IT MORE?

A DREAM

I asked for a job or position of importance. I was given a position, "Envoy".

I was introduced to a service envoy, who introduced me to his secretary of many years. She like me, was lonely, was over 800 years old and wanted to have children. Our children would be gifted like we were. The first child would be made, conceived or brought into existence. After the first child was born, we would have another child every five years. Strange dream.

We slept or spent the night together. There was no sex; she was a spirit without a body. In appearance, she looked like the three fallen angels, who visited me that night. I made the group, if they wished to stay, swear their love for Jesus Christ, and acceptance of His being, God, the Father Son and Holy Spirit.

Two of the three left and I baptized the other one, I poured water over his head, in the name of the Father, The Son (Jesus Christ), and the Holy Spirit.

I believed that I was granted the right, the responsibility to baptize those who desired it. Time passed and I was made aware that we do not baptize Fallen Angels. I prayed to God that noted we give man numerous chances. Angels, it seems to me, are higher up the ladder of acceptance than man.

Gabriel and Michael are examples of angels. I did not tell God he was wrong, but ask God to understand. The fallen angels are million, billion or maybe Googols. I am not informed or do not understand the reasons, but God says to forgive your enemy 70 x 7.

God is all-powerful, but He made man in his image and likeness. "I realize God is all-powerful" and feel that reducing the number of unhappy spiteful fallen angels would be good for all. They need be in love with God, the Father, Jesus Christ, the Son and the Holy Spirit.

One of three is not good, but a step forward. I still feel the "Baptized One" is a visitor in this home, "The Lord's Home", and I am the unhappy sinner servant who proposes this merger.

I am lost; I look for the Lord in my body and soul. I love Him truly and I am trying to love my enemy. I love God. May His will be done everywhere.

TO PRESIDENT BUSH

It has been months since Plato took his leave.
Plato is our resident groundhog. He will return we believe.

Summer died and autumn passed. Where to?
I don't know. The last two weeks we have had naught but snow.

January 20, 2005, President George W. Bush has been given a new four-year contract.
Ohio, a close call, backed Bush and expects jobs in return, tit for tit and tat for tat.

Bush is like Truman, debts he does pay.
Like California, he remembers those who stray.

He does not say much about it; George is a party man.
Free the world, democracy for all. Mr. President you are writing in the sand.

Socrates aspired to such a plan.
We have not the dollars for such a plan, but help we can.

"Police the world" is the cry.
And at each explosion our boys die

We also lost, it is noted, after seventeen years; the French gave up in Vietnam.
We were ready; we were tough. Good men died not in accordance with our plan

We finished the canal; after twelve years the French had given up.
We won that war against a mosquito … cost $10.00 a mosquito.

In each war we had endless dollars borrowed.
Money and brave men, we had a plenty. The money is spent and wives and mothers are sorrowed.

We cannot police the world as it is.
To attempt to do it; is all show biz.

Help we must and try we can.
The journey will be long and in accordance with a flexible plan.

The world is making progress with little supervision.
We must not try to occupy these countries, a non-military decision.

In many cases they have such a hard life … they just don't care.
They blow up women and children with joyous flair.

Try we should but walk softly, a military powerhouse not flaunted.
The dollars must be of a measurable amount; out treasury left undaunted.

Mr. President, at my age
I should be a sage.

I sit at the Veteran's table, magnificent seven.
We are respected as fighting men of the Army, Navy, & Air Force in days gone by.
Three of us are in our nineties; the others are not far behind.

We will soon pay our final bill.
Stand formation and march a final drill

If you want to help the Vets of World War II,
Do it today! Do your best; Congress is a slow working crew.

Today we should be asked for our advice.
We don't know all, realize the world is busy; remember us …be nice.

Mr. President, you, a wise man; ask both your parents for advice.
Your attention to family, all included is both wise and nice.

We seven helped you in Ohio
Work on Medicare and Social Security, a debt you owe.

Have a safe trip; the next four years will swiftly pass. You are in charge.
One at a time, the problems go away; the world is not so large.

January 27, 2005

THE SCENARIO -

Murele at Rue Morta
(690 Cooper Road, Westerville, OH)

It was the 31st day of July, 2005.
He (Ter loa) was fighting for his life.

Cancer was the aggressor and wanted Clyde's life.
His ex wife had a hit man's phone number and wishes him dead.

She pays Clyde support and is sorry they were wed.
Eighteen years married, now she wishes him dead.

The new threat wants Clyde to suffer the pains of starvation.
Who is she? Is she and that hit man one, a depreciation.

Designing ways, traps to catch the unfeeling vestige of murder
TRIP TO CORNELL

I was suddenly face to face with the "Arizona, I can't see a problem". I believe or I believed then — America is the "Land of the FREE and the Home of the Brave".

How did we accept the no admittance for blacks at our one and only municipal plunge. Yuma had days when the temperature would exceed 120 degrees. Hot! Hot! Hot!

My Father never mentioned the "problem" to me. He was appointed to the city recreation board and through his efforts; a swimming pool was built in the "colored" part of town.

Larry Ersorg, the Fraternity President, and I decided to drive through the south on the way to the Cornel Conference. We planned an extra week to visit the south.

We left Phoenix, Arizona in late April 1956. Things were in chaos and "set ins" and marches were beginning. That is they were in the process of a "coming out party". People were suddenly forced to admit "a problem existed".

Larry and I drove to New Orleans the first day. We were both Veterans and wanted to "do the town". We checked into a hotel, had a great dinner on Bourbon Street and didn't get back to the hotel until the sun was coming up.

August 5, 2005

FATHER CHARLES

With this small gift, we honor Thy Mother
In doing so, we honor The Father.
We hereby honor The Son
A noble endeavor for the Easter celebration
We thank Father Charles for his prayers and numerous insights.
In so doing, we honor God.
The Father, the Son and the Holy Spirit
The Son's gift to us was the gift of forgiven sin and redemption.
How does one repay the gift of life?
God would be happy, if we quit sinning. We can and must try.

MY LETTER TO THE LIVING

September 24, 2005

Note to the Partners of Paramount Senior Living at Westerville, Ohio

To: Food Service Coordinator

Re: Poor Food Service

Dear Coordinator:

I have lived at the "Outlook Manor" at Westerville, from March 2004 to March 2006. I have paid rent of $86,750.00 (eighty six thousand, seven hundred and fifty dollars). If I live ten more years, I will pay you another $450,000.000, at the current rate.

I am a polished gentleman and an excellent tenant (not perfect). I require very little care at present. I have suffered from Parkinson's for over twenty years. I have been fighting cancer the last two years. I suffer in silence and in private.

I graduated from Arizona State University, in Phoenix, Arizona, where I was an honor student. I was a graduate student at both ASU and the University of Southern California. I, also, studied advanced accounting at San Diego State University. I was a government agent for the U. S. Treasury Dept. for four years in Los Angeles, California. I was the auditor in charge for the Department of Defense in Santa Barbara, California for four years. I was the Senior Partner for a Certified Public Accounting Office in Santa Barbara. We had four CPA's in the office, and a staff of five support personnel. The last five years, I have written two books and over one hundred short stories and poems.

This background information is to establish my current health status. The Veterans Administration conducted six months of extensive tests in 2003. The VA declared me both physically and mentally competent. This testing was to qualify me for a deep brain operation. The operation should have reduced my tremor problems. The VA ran three complete body scans and two head scans. I may live ten to twenty more years. I am not senile, and have an excellent memory. My short term and long term memories are excellent.

The problem is food service; my major complaint is ice cream. Do not think me frivolous; this is a serious problem. It should be resolved in less than 10 minutes.

September 20, 2005, I requested ice cream. The server heard the request, but did not acknowledge it in any manner. I repeated the request fifteen minutes later. I requested ice cream a third time. I waited 45 minutes and did not receive the ice cream. The waiter would not confirm or deny my requests. This was repeated Wednesday, Thursday and Friday. I was ill Friday night and requested a dinner of a peanut butter and jelly sandwich and a dish of ice cream. I was given the regular dinner. I could not eat it. I was told "The staff did not have peanut butter and they would not give me the ice cream. The cancer treatment had caused my weight to drop from 170 to 135 pounds. I did not need to lose and must gain weight.

I called the nurse at 4:00, one hour before dinner. I had cramps and diarrhea. The nurse examined a black stool that I did not flush until she checked it.

The employees usually ignore my requests for ice cream. They know I will give up after 30 minutes. Ella told me to just ask.

Thursday, September 22, 2005, I requested ice cream four times over a 40 minute period. I was told, "They sent a waiter for it." Then, I was told, "They sent a waiter to check it out." Finally, I was told by Jim, "The ice cream was not unpacked and could not be served". (This was after I had waited 30 minutes.) A second waiter told me, "The only ones who they served ice cream were diabetics."

I went to the other dining room and checked. Bill, the retired Police Officer said, "They all were served a choice — chocolate, vanilla or pistachio nut ice cream. The ice cream dishes showed that most had been served the ice cream.

I checked with George and his wife; they were served in my dining room four servings of green pistachio nut ice cream for dinner that same night. George is not a diabetic.

It hurts for me to be told lies. The servers probably think all of us with "gray hair" are stupid and senile.

"You can tell them anything as they won't remember." I have just started my third book and I remember.

Ella told me a month ago, when I asked her what was the policy regarding the ice cream, "Clyde just ask for the ice cream." Ella never checked and Ella never received the ice cream.

I have been interested and would like to know the policy on ice cream. The $76,150, I paid for the last 19 months, should have covered the cost of ice cream.

Life is for the living, Service is what you should be GIVING! We share the same time and place. If you and I don't care we should give up the space.

Clyde C. Piatt

The Neurologist at St. Ann's Hospital prescribed the following: Every 1 ½ hours, while awake: one Sinemet, 25/100; At bedtime: one Sinemet, 50/200; Nightly at bedtime: one a day Seroquel, 25 mg.

Dr. Arora discussed with my son Cam that I should take: One Sinemet 25/100 every 2 hours. This is a 50% reduction for me, and I have been managing my medication for 18 years. They also discussed that I am suffering withdrawal from Sinemet. I experience lots of pain from leg cramps and convulsions. I also have kidney pain rating 8 on a 10 point scale, and fears shutdown of my kidneys and possible liver shutdown. I "blew" my prostrate when the Sinemet stopped.

I currently fear a stroke or heart attack. I am under extensive pressure, suffering severe shakes and leg convulsions. I have been refused aspirin that I have taken the past 20 years (one a day). I am suffering extensive mental pain due to the Sinemet reduction. He suggested a 25% reduction as it would not be as much a shock to my neurological system. Dr. Arora and Cam denied my request.

I shake too much and can't hold a fork and must eat in my room. I can't stand up four or five times a day, until Sinemet is absorbed after taking pills. I become frozen with full body shakes. I need not suffer. A 25% reduction, 2 weeks after would have cut the pain in half.

I have taken Minocyclene for 30 years. Why have we stopped? My skin condition is worse. I am weak in the legs and arms. I cannot even lift covers over me. I am in pain in my legs and lower back. The right side rates 8 out of 10 on a regular basis. I become frozen at times, especially in the legs and my back becomes bowed, I am often unable to brush my teeth and sometimes my whole right side just freezes. I am also experiencing blurred vision; I cannot see the side of my face in the mirror. I am writing smaller and less legibly, am always tired and exhausted and more often than not, hungry. The tremors even prevent urination, at times.

October 19, 2005, Thursday

November 28, 2005
DIRECTORS, OUTLOOK MANOR
COOPER ROAD, WESTERVILLE, OHIO

To: Directors, Officers and Employees

Scope: Many of the Residents, who are able to complain, are sick of your employee lack of leadership and sick of your employee insubordination, mean and uncaring ways. The owners are negligent and should make themselves available to residents.

You have many problem areas. I have been a resident for two years and two months. I am ready to leave. I have had Parkinson's for twenty years and I suffer day and night. I have cancer and have suffered for the past two and a half years with it. Two years ago, the Doctor gave me one to three years to live.

It is possible we could correct these problems at Outlook. Many of us will never be happy again. You, the owners, are responsible and you must care. God does not take kindly to people who abuse the old and the sick. It is a serious sin.

I am paying $3,700 a month and have paid over $80,000.00 rent. The food quality and presentation has improved in the past two months. Your purchase procedures are practiced poorly. You run out of jam, jelly, butter, crackers, peanut butter, ice cream, sugar, juice, coffee, hot chocolate mix, bread, etc. We have not had fresh rolls for a week. You send leg of lamb; it is old, not good and a joke. I requested mint jelly and it was served once. It is now available with leg of lamb. You have us fill out spread order forms and, many times, run out of product.

The Veterans table ordered six steaks. Our table was often the last served and that night, we ordered six steaks; they served everyone else, but we were not served steaks. We had waited over thirty minutes, before the server placed our second choice. They should correct the steak orders. Many servers do a "great job and care". You have forty per cent who do not care. When you ask them a question, they give you a blank stare, do not acknowledge the resident in any manner. I call it the "dumb stare". I have requested the same item three times before receiving acknowledgement of the request. I have seen it happen fifty times to others.

The "dumb stare" is used by aids. They ignore cries for help — screaming elderly ladies. When some of us NOT SO SICK ask them to help, the aid pulls the "dumb stare" act.

We know there are people who "cry wolf", demand attention and are difficult. The "cry wolf" is sick and must be cared for. We, who are "not so sick" are suffering, the screams cause us concern and anxieties.

We have run out of bread, out of milk, out of creamers, out of ice cream, out of peanut butter since I have been here. The past three days, we have not had sweet rolls of any kind.

I have lost sixty-five pounds, since I have been sick. I am anemic and need extra calories. I have been given the "dumb stare" treatment, ignored and lied to — "We don't have any ice cream. The package has not been opened.

The last note, I wrote to the Directors was not acknowledged by the owners. If I can find their addresses, I will mail a copy of this letter.

Please realize, I am a senior citizen and I am not senile. I have an I Q of 160 +. I am a published author. I have an excellent memory, both short term and long term. I have been examined by three physicians in the past six months. I will no longer accept the "dumb stare" response. I love people and have not created problems intentionally.

The nurse, who refuses to give me two Tylenol tablets, will comply with the doctor's instructions, and give me two, not one tablet, or I will write a complaint letter to the directors and staff.

Almost all of the nurse's are skilled, caring people who do a great job. The two or three nurses who give me the "dumb stare" approach, I will report.

I believe that with a few changes Outlook Manor can improve and be a first rate home for the sick, tired, old and dying patients herein — "Who Need Care"

Sincerely,

Clyde C. Piatt

P.S.I am a CPA who had clients who ran "rest homes" in Texas, California, Arizona and Nevada. I was in charge of a CPA firm with a staff of nine, when I retired.

I am finishing my second book. I submitted my first book to a New York publisher, two weeks ago. There are plans for a third book about elderly care, The "Golden Years", A Grimm Fairy Tale.

The people who deliver the meals to the sick in their rooms have intentionally lost or thrown away my meal order. I no longer order room service. I drag myself to the dining room, if I can. If I am too sick, I will go without the meal.

They parked my meal and "forgot" my order. They refused an order for Peanut Butter and Jelly (out of Peanut Butter). I would trace the meal and received my meal late. I complained, but never heard the results.

Shake, stutter, write poorly, but I am not throwing in the towel. Give your employees a pat on the back. Let them know their work is appreciated. "I was employee of the month." Give them a special parking place for the month.

AGREEMENT:

The nurse who refused to give medication prescribed by the doctor will be questioned and may be dismissed.

Nurse instructions regarding Clyde C. Piatt, Room # 501, effective December 25, 2005: Medications will not be delivered more than 15 minutes late. If delivery is more than 15 minutes late, the nurse will write a letter explaining non-compliance to doctor. The nurse will deliver medication to Clyde if he is awake or if he is sleeping or napping. Clyde may alternately pick up medication 15 minutes before due.

8:00 a.m.: Sinemet 25/100 mg, Sinemet 50/200 mg, Ferdovel .25 mg, 1 Aspirin, 2 Tylenol 500mg or 3 325 mg. 9:30 a.m.: Sinemet 25/100 — not extended relief. 11:00 a.m.: Sinemet 25/100. 12:30 p.m.: Sinemet 25/100. 2:00 p.m.: Sinemet 25/100. 3:30 p.m.: Sinemet 25/100. 5:00 p.m.: Sinemet 25/100, Sinemet 50/200. 6:30 p.m.: Sinemet 25/100. 8:00 p.m.: Sinemet 25/100, Sinemet 50/200, Seroquel .25, Tylenol 2 or 3 tablets. 9:30 p.m.: Sinemet 25/100. 11:00 p.m.: Sinemet 25/100. 12:30 a.m.: Sinemet 25/100. 2:00 a.m.: Sinemet 25/100. 3:30 a.m.: Sinemet 25/100. 5:00 a.m.:Sinemet 25/100. 6:30 a.m.: Sinemet 25/100. Clyde may also receive ½ of Sinemet 25/100 two times a day (up to Clyde and not up to nurse). Pills late will be given to Clyde. Pill times will not be changed by nurse.

Signed by Doctor
Signed by Clyde C. Piatt

JERRY'S PARADE

President Gerald Ford's Funeral — January 2, 2006

Very nice, strong and wise,
He headed us, eased our cries.

Friend and foe, formal and staid,
Prayed and honored Jerry's last parade.

We all who cared, knew him well,
Not a flamboyant leader.

All of us were embarrassed by "Watergate"
President Ford exposed all, apologized,

And asked us to have faith.
He was an outstanding, courageous, honest man of state.

My Lord, God of all, He will serve you well!
Clyde C. Piatt

HE WANTS IN

I am tired, I am sad.
Though not mad, I have been had.

You try to smile, gild covers the bile.
The truth is a crocodile. Mean, unafraid, master of guile

Love the family,
Beware of the dog tied to the tree

If you pet him, he may stay.
Best to leave him alone unless he can pay.

Don't answer his calls.
He can walk, so what if he falls.

We have our own lives to live — "Sigh, let him die."
If you give an inch Auntie says, you will be had, let him cry.

Though love, no alms or charity for the sick,
Auntie said, it is all a trick,
Don't open the door; he is slick.

ENJOY THE DAY

The sun, our nearest star, is nine light minutes away.
Alpha Centuri, the next star is 4.3 light years and that is a long way.

Today is cold, misty rain and I am not at my emotional best.
My bones ache and my feet are damp, cramped and cold.

Not one in a thousand know the size of the heavens above.
There are fewer still; who realize the reason we have dove.

Often in life, my mind is in space and I must wrestle it back so I may save face.
The vastness of space is no greater than that of the mind, which is housed in a rather small space.

Right or wrong is not always the most important part of being.
How we arrived at the answer is, the insight we need, as important as seeing.

Do your research work thoroughly and do not be in a rush.
To examine an exquisite jewel or an exquisite rose, don't be in a rage to crush.

Let beauty be as is and as peaceful as the dove.
Beauty has run away, it is true and it was love.

Thank the power that holds sway.
Be thankful, you had beauty even for a day.

LOCKED IN

The end, and the beginning is lost
Why Parkinson's for seventeen years of pain and the cost

I have not been forced to bankruptcy yet
Tomorrow's worries I will not fret

Two weeks in the "assisted living home"
Loneliness has me, but alive; it is cold, but it is not HOME

Cancer is here, not wanted, loaded down with FEAR
Seventeen months of chemo is nothing to cheer

Radio Active Iodine 125 cooks twenty-four hours a day in my Prostate gland
Seeds they planted, 110 in number; at times I am too weak to stand

My urine smells life sulfur, rotten egg
My other excretions smell like roasted flesh

I have suffered enough and told the Doctor
Doctor said, "Cancer". I asked him the killing time

He said, "If you do not fight, you have one to three years."
The way I feel today, alone with my fears, pain, loneliness, throw in the towel with no fears

January 16, 2006

P.S. I know what day it is and my brain appears to be working.

PIATT DREAMS

I sometimes have dreams. They sometimes make sense, but not always. Often they are not realistic. Sometimes I am afraid and feel threatened, yet sometimes they are happy. I pray a lot in my dreams and ask, pray to God to not allow the devil or his associates to invade the space I look after for God, the Father, the Son and the Holy Spirit (God!). I sometimes have spirits appear during these dreams. They move seldom and speak never. Their mouths do not move, but somehow, I hear them. They do not answer me directly, but somehow, I receive messages. The beautiful lady in white and blue left the message, “I should not be afraid”.

On two or three occasions, I was visited by 20 to 30 spirits, all ages, baby to adult. These spirits do not identify themselves. I demand they be Christians, accept Jesus Christ as God, believe in the trinity; they must accept Christ as their Savior, the Son of God and our Lord. Three men in dark suits, clean, pressed appeared. They did not speak. They had square jaws and an animal look, not so much did I see the animal, but I sensed what could have been a look that I thought had the appearance of a goat-like profile. They were not ugly, were well mannered, but I was on guard.

I preached to them, asked them to raise their colors. I told them to pray to God, accept my terms or leave. I explained I would have to leave the final decision to God. Jesus would have to grant me approval. I told the three God was a forgiving God. I thought if they were fallen angels and repented, accepted Jesus Christ as God’s Son and their God, He would probably forgive them. Two left and there was one.

He did not speak, but informed me that he wanted God's forgiveness and accepted my terms. I baptized him pouring water over his head, "I baptize you in the name of the Father, the Son and the Holy Spirit." I have not seen any of the three again. I have felt the presence of the baptized spirit.

One dream, I told the Lord, through prayer, that I was sick and alone; I needed a job, wanted to serve God as his paperboy or clerk, servant, as I needed a purpose. I met a spirit who was an aid for God's work; she was 800 or more years old, like me, and she was lovely. She wanted children. God's work group checked with (I assume Christ) God and they seemed to have approved my marriage to this spirit. She had no body and was a spirit, but somehow could have children with me - one child to be born every five years. I was to go to work for God as an envoy! I would travel extensively and be a negotiator. I would not return for 10 years — Inform my son!

The dream was crystal clear. She had features and dressed not unlike the three visitors.

She was working as a fund raiser at the hospital, where I was taken for observation. She did not talk to me. Nodded three or four times, did not want me to talk to her, but seemed concerned with my illness. I blew her a few kisses. She made me feel emancipated. She indicated that she could smuggle me out and we could leave the hospital if I was a prisoner. She never said a word.

February 15, 2006

Compounds Could Slow Parkinson's Disease

By LAURAN NEERGAARD, Associated Press Medical Writer ~AP February 23, 2006

An antibiotic and a muscle-related compound are leading candidates for a major government study of whether certain compounds could slow the worsening of Parkinson's disease. A pilot study, unveiled Thursday, suggests the two — the antibiotic minocycline and creatine, a substance produced in muscle tissue — may have some benefit. It's far too early for patients to seek the pills, stressed Dr. Diane Murphy, who oversees Parkinson's research at the National Institutes of Health, which funded the work. But in the study of 200 patients in the earliest stages of the disease — they didn't yet require medication for its symptoms — those who took either of the two pills didn't seem to decline quite as rapidly as those given a dummy pill, scientists said Thursday at Parkinson's meeting in Washington. The compounds are thought to lessen a type of cellular stress or fight inflammation that may damage cells.

About 1.5 million Americans have Parkinson's disease, which gradually destroys brain cells that produce dopamine, a chemical crucial for the cellular communication that controls muscle movement. As dopamine levels drop, symptoms increase: tremors in the arms, legs and face; periodically stiff or frozen limbs; slow movement; impaired balance and coordination. Standard treatments are to replace lost dopamine with the drug levodopa, and a brain implant to control tremors. Both work for a while, but can't stop the disease's inevitable march.

So NIH's National Institute of Neurological Disorders and Stroke is on a hunt for drugs that might protect patients' remaining dopamine-producing cells, a so-called neuroprotector. The Holy Grail would be a simple, easy-to take pill that would lower the risk of worsening Parkinson's much like an aspirin a day can lower people's risk of heart attacks. "We're looking for the aspirin of Parkinson's disease," is how Murphy puts it. "We don't have a drug like that right now, and we don't know of such a drug," she cautions.

That's where the pilot study comes in. NIH asked Parkinson's specialists for a list of potential neuroprotective compounds — substances that could enter the brain and seemed promising in animal studies. From an initial list of 60, they settled on four to pilot-test. The minocycline and creatine results are first in, published in the journal Neurology online this week and announced Thursday at the World Parkinson Congress. Now being analyzed is a similar study on the dietary supplement coenzyme Q-10 or CoQ10 and an experimental drug thought to help repair damaged nerves.

Next up, NIH plans to test the top candidates in a large study to prove whether any of them truly work. Minocycline is a prescription-only antibiotic, but creatine is available in dietary supplements. Murphy cautioned that over-the-counter preparations of creatine or CoQ10 may not be the same strengths as are under study.

GOD'S MESSAGE

I at least heard you and understood your message. Your delivery was excellent. The Bible is clear, help feed the beggar and you assist God. Jesus Christ is pleased.

I was a Treasury Agent, U. S. Treasury, in Los Angeles, California. The office was at 1031 South Broadway. Fear was dispensed by drunks and drug addicts; some gave alms, others declined. They were the "get a job" advisors. Some said, "Many are not in need." Many are hungry, broke and alone. I don't care if I help some ingrate. If one in three needs my change — I am pleased!

You are a gifted speaker. Don't condemn the handicapped, who on his dying bed or the sidewalks of L.A., because he stutters, is confused and does not remember the words.

You leered "PERFECT". Fear was your apparent reason; you were defending confession. My speech is broken. My memory is intact. I am a Parkinson's-suffering man, who can't say a perfect act of contrition. I have suffered from Parkinson's for twenty years. But, I can say to Jesus, "MY LORD", I believe you are the Son of God, my Master, forgive my sins; I love you." God, the Father, Son and Holy Spirit would grant my forgiveness.

If faced with death, why try? I can't say a "Perfect Act of Contrition". It would be a waste of time to say. I am sorry, Jesus; please forgive me. I love you!"

I received the last rights three months ago. The Father absolved me of all my sins. My Parish Priest said I should confess these sins. He seemed to say, “The absolution by last rights is not acceptable. It is a simple question.”

April 3, 2006

May 8, 2006

Jon, I write to be heard
One day, my labors will be classic.

Van Gogh sold one painting to his brother
A life difficult, lost, but later discovered.

His paintings now sell for 5, 10, 50 million each,
Artistic rewards are lost until found by a scholar who sees.

The “Rosetta Stone” a treasure made, lost, found.
It opened the door of knowledge for many.

My writings are and will be important to one.
I see things not many people see.

SHADY ACRES

The "last stop" is a Rest Home
The home of Angels

For the old and those taking an early flight
We won't forget your name

Your friends are few
Three or four, including the "Lady in Red", a Jew

Two Catholics and an Agnostic one
Quit crying; it is done

Alluvial & Willow, NE Corner
A Baked field in Fresno's California sun

I lived there for over a year, overstayed my welcome
Had two sons when I arrived

OHIO

This morning is cold — cold — cold
The sun has delayed the day and time is old

We are not getting any younger
September was mild, it goes and so goes the summer

The year is on the run, my third year in Ohio
Three operations in Ohio plus one in California before moving here

I am without energy and low on patience
The food server said, “I used to be a nice guy” — past tense

I am a “NICE GUY” — love people — don’t make me cry
You did promise coffee “in a second”
Ken waited 32 minutes and no breakfast, but you try.

I asked you, “Are going to bring Ken his food?”
You did not answer.
I asked you if you were going to bring Ken breakfast?

You answered naught.
I asked, “If you were bringing Ken’s breakfast?”
A blank stare was all I got.

You served his plate 35 minutes late

You treated me like fish bait

No show of remorse and no sorry
Anger only, I worry

Better days be with you
I am sorry too!

September 20, 2006

THE ELDERLY LADY & THE COFFEE

Yesterday, September 24, 2006, an elderly lady, age 93, in a wheelchair, was angry because she had received no coffee. She stretched as far as she could reach; pulled down a full pot of coffee from the rack next to the Veterans table of six men. She was about to set the coffee pot in her lap. It would have burned her and she would have spilled the full pot in her lap.

McDonald's paid a million dollars on a coffee spill. Clyde grabbed the pot after yelling at a waiter three times. The situation was serious. We need some guidelines. Employees should not ignore pleas. Get some complaint slips.

September 27, 2006

They put a pot on our table.
Coffee it was to be.
What it was? It smelled like pee.
Ella checked it out for me.
She thought it was funny
I am afraid to complain
Not funny; insane
I try to be honest — I try!
My complaints, I put in writing.
You think it funny, but you do not put it in writing.
The coffee pot — an important note was ignored.
Probably a laughable joke to you, too

THE DIRTY COFFEE POT

The coffee pot was filthy. It was not clean; it was caked with food from a past day. The staff said it was pasta. What difference does it make? It could have been oatmeal, chili, macaroni, spaghetti, etc. Dirty food particles are ugly, can hide germs. I seldom get diarrhea or related problems. Why do you make a point? I did not get sick, therefore — you are trying to tell me that dirty crud is acceptable on dishes you eat off or use? Dirty on the outside leads me to suspect worse on the inside. This dirty pot on top of yesterday's dirty pot is not funny — not A.O.K. to me.

I have been in a fight, for two and a half years, demanding coffee be served me within fifteen minutes after seating. Most restaurants serve coffee in one to five minutes after seating. The servers did not like being ordered to serve the coffee. When you ask for coffee, they used to say, "You will have to wait until we serve all the people breakfast.

I have paid rent of $210,000.00 to you and I am ready to leave this place. There are two or three who may go with me. If you prefer dirty dishes, continue on, but I will not eat out of dirty dishes or drink coffee out of pots that have not been washed. You make me feel like I am sick, senile or demented. I have been checked by five psychiatrists and 28 neurologists in the last twenty years. I am not demented or psychotic. I have excellent memory — short and long term.

I like people and will help those in need if able. I have called the police twice in the past ten years. I told them that my call was not an emergency. You ignored my plea to take care of the ninety year old lady, in the wheelchair, with the coffee pot in her hand. The pot was about to be spilled in her lap. When I yelled for assistance, your employees ignored my plea. I was incapacitated by Parkinson's in an off mode. I jumped up and rescued the elderly lady at a substantial risk to myself. You did nothing — not even a thank you. I wrote this note because the woman mentioned is ignoring the issue.

These people need help and care. I have reported twelve distress calls in the past year. They were late night falls. It takes as long as thirty minutes for calls to be checked. I shake, freeze and walk, but I try.

SERVICE BUZZER

We are told that the buzzer will bring help. We assume that means within three to five minutes. If a resident has a heart attack, chances are he or she will die. Thirty minutes response time is common. I know of several times an hour and several cases with no reply after an hour. You advertise twenty-four hour nurse service. Residents should be told to sign up for a life support service that does not leave you on the floor. You have a computer program for control purposes. You do not follow up and are probably communally negligent, too. I freeze up, can't move and have three minutes, five minutes, fifteen minutes, thirty minutes, and no response calls. What is your policy?

We had a tornado watch. The nurse in charge told me to go to my room. It is an upstairs room with a window. Experts advise going to a downstairs room with no windows. You advise that going to an UPSTAIRS ROOM WITH WINDOWS was O.K. You would be the first to go. Adopt a Policy.

I was ordered loudly by an attendant, "Go to your room!" No questions were asked. I went to my room, did not know if I should stay three minutes or three days. I could have had a HEART ATTACK.

ELDERLY ABUSE

The only advice you gave me, was to quit picking
You did not have time to treat my illness
Be it real or fantasy
You wasted no time in calling and probing
You choked when I requested the material you cut out.
It was more important for you to destroy the evidence
It would or could have proved you right.
It may well be you are a fool.
The mental problem you suggest, could have been put to rest
For this elderly man seeking an end to his quest.
For the truth is elusive
Hidden, tortured and murdered by your care,
Elderly abuse

THE FATHER, THE SON

I was sighted, yet, I did not see the clear bursts of lightning, I see
The trees grouped together were a forest
I saw the forest, but failed the test
Miracles, like lightning are many
Not announcements, no thunder or cymbals
The righteous man who questioned God for letting him down
God had sent two rescue squads and a helicopter
The man, three-times refused God's help
How many minutes have we witnessed?
We never forget prayers unanswered
Many years ago, my best friend was lost
I did not know how I would find him
A long drive to his apartment and many hours of searching
Tired and not thinking clearly
I drove to the University where he was a student
It was a large campus, over ten thousand students
I did a lot of praying
Was a miracle in the plan?
For a few minutes, I drove around the campus
The sun was disappearing and night was fast approaching
It had been a long day
I was low, distraught, tired and hungry, feet of clay
He must have directed me
One last drive through the main entrance gate
A young emaciated man sat under the tree

Shoes off, lost and alone; it was he
Was this a miracle?
It was arranged by He; not an accident
The father and the son cried
And I know so did He
The three of us prayed together
God had made all the arrangements, His treat, no advanced seating
The prayer meeting did not last long
We all remember the time and place
We thank Him for His Grace
We often forget the miracles
We receive or witness
How is it possible?
I suspect the devil's hand; his ways are rotten
We must try harder
This father and son thank God
For care and His grace

I had four difficult trips to the VA Hospital in San Francisco. I traveled alone, in a U.S.

Government van; with leg cramps and in excruciating pain. The trips were for testing to qualify me for the deep brain surgery program.

I was ill and was released from St. Agnes Hospital in Fresno the day before. I was operated on for prostrate problems. The hospital was a lonely place. There was no one to stick up for me. I told the doctor that I suffered delusions, nightmares and terrible agony if given pain medicine or narcotics.

I was scheduled for a Friday morning surgery. I woke up in a private room. I inquired about the operation. The doctor mumbled, "You are doing fine." It was an operation without an outside incision.

It was late Sunday before I was informed, "the operation was not performed." No one would tell a sick old man, with a broken heart, that he would never be put "back together again".

I did not cry. A sinner must pay for his sins and God must be angry. Job was a righteous man and he was tortured many times. No one would tell me what transpired. I was a lonely, sick old man. A beautiful angel, named Heather, from Mexico, told me that I had ripped out four intravenous tubes and tried to rip out the urine drain tube.

The day after they cancelled the operation, I was admitted to St. Agnes Hospital in Fresno,

California. I was in too much pain. I was in the hospital ten days; had not one solitary visitor. The days were long. After the operation was done, the next day, they had given me a pain shot, after I had explained to them in detail that I could not take the pain shots.

I moved to Ohio to stay with my son, Cameron, for six months. I have lived at Outreach Manor for three years. Time still flies. Cameron told me that I was invited over for brunch (10:00-11:45). He would pick me up and return me. As quite often happened, I was sick that day and cancelled. I have cancelled many times, because I was ill.

December 23, 2006

Not many remember the date, but it was February 11 in 1934. There will be fewer who remember the day next year. I am sick, broke, but not busted. Each month I feel a little better. They are small steps, but it is progress. Money is important to me, but only to eat and pay my medical bills. I do not waste it. I resent having my lack of funds being blown up. I made it through my divorces and they were expensive.

Sarah loved me or used me. She worked the twelve years she was married before me. She took a ten year vacation after she married me. I have paid $200,000 to $300,000 in medical bills the past twenty years. In a pension plan, I would have $600,000 to $900,000. My bills were paid. I paid my first wife Roberta "Bobbie" alimony by giving her most of our property. I have paid my way in life. There will be no change in the next few years.

Cameron was reimbursed all his expenses, I think. I had the presence of mind to borrow the money for the divorce and move. I do feel guilty about Sarah. She lied to me; her Mother told me Sarah would take care of me. She said, “Sarah is loyal, she will take care of you”.

NO NAME, NO ONE TROUBLE IN MY CASE, PARKINSON'S IS TROUBLE

Trouble came from nowhere, uninvited and unwanted
It was received and accepted, hidden by the intended undaunted

It was dealt with in life's shadow world for many long years
It was a form of denial true, but not made out of fear

A man's world is often a closed secret place
Where pride, arrogance and determination set the pace

We hide our ignorance and our doubts even from ourselves
Ever seeking the pot of gold hidden by the elves

The pot contains glory, esteem of self, lofty position as well as gold
Trouble is ever waiting to pounce on the self-seeking, young or old

Trouble saps your strength as well as your desire to deceive
It is time to expose your trouble to those you should appease

Intelligent ones will tell you, that they knew you had met trouble
The little changes, and the big bad years before, burst your bubble

Your secrets were not secrets hidden by you in fear

In the early years they were shared by those you hold dear

If trouble seeks you, uninvited and unwanted, and finds you
Get his name, study his past, analyze and test him too

Run up your flag, grab your staff, and prepare for battle
Put trouble in a cage, display it, and give it a great rattle

Family and friends will join you in stride
For they know that, from trouble you cannot hide

In time, the road will be shown to those whose feet are not clay
Have faith, be strong of heart; He will show the way

Smile and laugh, you need laughter now more than ever before
The joke is not on you; trouble is in trouble for evermore

Modern science and research are making giant strides every day
Trouble may soon leave you; a cure is on the way

I have suffered the pain and terrible mental stress of "The Shaky Palsy" for twenty years. I have not escaped any of the torture associated with the disease. I pray to my God for release from the pain, but all I receive is more pain.

Jesus Christ prayed for release from His suffering. He knew everything; he would be tortured, public whipping, thorns driven into his head, spit from his people, the Jews, ridicule, a loving Mother, who was forced to watch, friends who denied knowing him, huge nails driven through his hands and feet, and He, "God forgave them".

I, a sinner, have been brave for twenty years. I have suffered more than twenty years, and I am spent. If another man gave this disease to my son, I would try to kill him.

I suffer terrible leg cramps for six to eight hours at a time. I thought the extent of pain was limited, but in the last month, they found a new way to torture me. I drop off to sleep, exhausted and the devils wake me up in 45 minutes to 1 ½ hours. I am frozen, unable to move a finger. I can talk, yell, but no one hears.

It requires every bit of strength to move a finger, then a hand, then a leg; — bit by bit, I am able to move. I slap my legs and move them with my hands. I toss and turn, exercise my mental power to push my legs off the bed, moves of ¼ inch at a time. With super human effort, I work my feet to the floor. The legs still frozen, I move a toe. The process takes 15 — 30 minutes and I am rewarded with a stilt use of my legs to fall forward to a heavy stuffed chair, on which I fall. I soon walk. What a joy!

This happened every other night at first; soon it was twice a night. The sleep time is now less than one hour. It is HELL and I know things never get better with Parkinson's. They only get worse.

This is not the only curse, but it is one mean one. The Lord Jesus probably knew his fate from the instant of birth or before. He suffered mentally His whole life. He did ask the Father to be saved from the pain.

I am not strong enough to accept the torture and pain and pray it is lifted from me. I know and love the Father, but cannot stand the tortured feeling that Ike was not treated fairly.

Parkinson's is an ever-changing disease. It cripples you a day at a time and is without pity. There is a day coming when it will be treatable. It is not far off. We have used five year periods for the last twenty years. We are making progress. You can read this book and you will be disturbed by one man's story. A story of love lost. The primary cause is Parkinson's. I have included the pain and suffering as it is part of my life's story.

The ultimate end of my marriage is probably a direct result of the disease, too. It is sad, but many long term marriages between

Parkinson's partners end up in divorce. It would be nice if those dissolutions were the result of friendly agreements. They are more of the result of bottled up hate. The resulting dissolution is often a battle fought without a victor.

My trial is not over and will continue until the Parkinson's disease is settled. I have listed my major problems and did not try to disguise my real and imagined problems. I believe that I am still capable of writing and though ravaged by Parkinson's, not yet demented. We shall see.

The writing is difficult to read and requires a great effort to write. I am trying. The new

Parkinson's has shown remarkable progress at Ohio State University, Columbus, Ohio.

Gene Therapy inserted into the brain by a virus. It has improved muscle controls by 25 to 30% and by a whopping 65% in a few isolated cases.

Parkinson's is a progressive disease, has infected about one million Americans. We sufferers have tremors of the fingers, hands, arms, legs. It can affect the whole body. You may notice small legible handwriting, slurred speech, reduced ability to speak, problems swallowing, etc. Last night, I awoke in a frozen state, went through my ritual of working a finger until it thawed; freeing my toes from the frozen state, one at a time; freeing a foot, a leg, sliding the cover until I free fall to the floor, crawl until I can crawl up a chair. In the end, I am standing, not very steady. Then it is time to slide my feet forward and miracle time — I am walking.

If I could afford a male nurse, I would not have to do this myself. In the meantime, I will push, crawl, fall and drag myself.

The Neurosurgeon assisted by the most advanced computer images and surgical techniques is implanting a hair-sized wire deep in the brain. They connect this to a battery pack in the upper chest. This is turned on a three to five volt charge is used to zap the sick cells. It works, but in its own way.

I suffered severe leg cramps for over twenty years. They disappeared after the operation. It was a pleasant surprise. Three months later, they returned. The tremors have gone and to date they have not returned.

Ali R. Rezai is in charge of the Cleveland Clinic Neuro surgery Department. He is a very highly recognized brain surgeon. The Cleveland Clinic is a world-class hospital with thirty-six thousand on the payroll. The active staff, involved with my operation, is outstanding. Dr. Rezai told me he was tempted to sew me up without finishing the operation. It seems that while under the knife, you must remain awake to talk the surgeons through your brain. I had called Dr. Rezai a devil. I have shown by past reactions to narcotics and other drugs, I go nuts. I told the Doctor that it was not me. I loved, respected, and had a great faith in his ability. The devil made me do it. I trust he was kidding. I apologized to the whole department — a devil indeed — more like unto an angel. This team is probably the best in the world and I would recommend the Cleveland Clinic to all the candidates for the operation.

I have been to thirty neurosurgeons in the past twenty years and I am an expert. I was having the operation performed in San Francisco, California, two years before. They had the four-post crown in place, blood dripped from the four posts and I ordered the operation stopped. They removed the crown and I checked out.

Dr, Rezai can walk on water, if he wants to. He was referred by Dr. Mahlon DeLong, Head of Neurology, at Emory University. Dr. Rezai worked for DeLong at Emory, for over ten years and at Johns Hopkins over ten years, before being hired away from Emory. He has the number one surgeon in the world working for him. It is Ali R. Rezai, himself.

Parkinson's disease is incurable. The researchers are making progress and will come up with a cure. It may be one year or more, but will be within the next ten years.

Michael J. Fox used five years in most of his battle. With workers like Michael and Mohammed Ali, we will win.

They are finding new approaches that are indicating a new approach in the antibiotic Minocyclene, Creatine, virus-loaded cells planted in the brain directly and standard treatment include Levadopa and a brain implant to control tremors

The results are promising, but stop working in some patients. I have taken Sinemet for 21 years and still receive a benefit from Sinemet. I take 16 — 100 mg. Sinemet and 25 — 25 Levadopa pills a day. The Cleveland Clinic operated on my brain in March 2007 and my tremors have decreased by 90%. The effects of the operation are not controllable. I was pleased, when I found my leg cramps and spasms had disappeared, but was very sad when they returned three months later.

It has been 9 months since the operation and I am still tremor free.

April 30, 2006

Dear Marian and Sir Cloud:

I still try but feel lowly
The days go slowly

Time has not been my friend
I am in a hurry for time to end

I think of you all
Miss you and pray you don't fall

The golden years are a rip
I think I have missed the HAPPY TRIP

It is time — put on the warrior's paint
War on age, fight to kill, don't faint

A broken heart mends
Find a friend

Build a fire, dance, sing
The God's will smile; bells will ring

The smoke will tell God; we are not having fun
We need to hear, to see, to feel, to taste; we need to be young!

A MAN'S CHILDREN ARE HIS BEST INVESTMENTS.

HAPPY FATHER'S DAY

EVER CONSIDER ROUNDING OUT
YOUR PORTFOLIO WITH SOME
FLORIDA SWAMP LAND AND AN
OPTION ON THE BROOKLYN BRIDGE?

Dear Dad,

We're both looking forward to seeing you and Sarah soon.

I hope you enjoy the book. I haven't read it, but I read TheFirm and The Pelican Brief. He's an o.k. writer. I looked for that author you always read, but I couldn't find one.

Work hard, real busy, high stress, but I think it will get easier soon.

Happy Father's Day
Love,

Cam & Becky

POSTLOGUE

By Joyce Dusenbury

The calls and meeting have done wonders in relieving the lifelong stress for me

Whatever is best for you and your family, from further pain I hope you all will be free

BECAUSE YOU ARE YOU

It was spring 2007; I met a very special man
I interviewed him for activities — sure as I can

Not knowing what a life he led
Until later, after some time had sped

While I was at the front desk, he said,
"Do you know anyone who could do some typing for me?"
I replied, "I could do some typing for you, Clyde."

Within a few days; there was much typing to do
You didn't tell me a book was coming through

A few days later, I asked your deadline
Two weeks from Tuesday was your reply; I whined

Later when I asked if this was true, you said, "You asked for a date
So I gave it to you!" You smiled! Thank God! It would have been late!

As I have typed your stories and words of wisdom
I have gained a great respect for your intellect

When we had the social club near the fireplace
You shared your words deep from your heart

Your Mom, on her deathbed said,
"Your Dad was the kindest and best man she ever met
And you are just like him."

I totally agree with her and yet, I never met your Dad.
These precious words from you really made me glad.

Clyde, somewhere in your words you said,
"What do I have to offer?"

You have a beautiful, deep, caring, loving heart
And you always have right from the start

You have an incredible mind and brain
And great success, you have attained

You are a strong man to have endured all
That you have come through — even with the falls

You have a God given talent to write
And with all these words, it is so right

To share your stories is such a gift
For the rest of the world — "YOU ARE THE GIFT"

And you definitely are not a toad
You are a prince with a heavy load

I pray for you with every day
And keep you in my thoughts along the way

Thank you, Clyde, for being you
You'll have your dreams when they are due.

Joyce Dusenbury, August 31, 2007

SNOWMEN FOR CLYDE AND CALEB

Clyde, it is a joy to see your eyes,
When your precious little Grandson, Caleb, arrives.

Caleb, your Grandpa is a sweet and gentle man,
So come to visit him whenever you can.

Caleb, you are a precious little boy;
Your special Grandpa for you to enjoy.

You bring great love into his heart
So from his heart do not depart.

He lights up when you are around,
Even though sometimes, you don't make a sound.

Now you and Grandpa have something to share,
A wonderful bond, no one can compare.

Enjoy these matching blankets 'tis true
Stay happy and healthy, and don't be blue.

The snowmen on your quilts are fun,
As they won't melt away with the warm morning sun.

So enjoy your cozy warm quilts
Made with love, as they were built.

Joyce Dusenbury, October 17, 2007

AUTHOR'S SPECIAL ACKNOWLEDGEMENTS

Thank you to Joyce Dusenbury, for the extensive editing, typing, and assembly of this book. Joyce shared with me, many times, what an honor it was to help with my story.

As Joyce read and typed my words, her enthusiasm grew, because this book will help so many Parkinson's patients and their families to understand this disease and learn what to expect in their future. She is very dedicated to helping others and she is thrilled I am sharing my story.

I decided, the first time I met Joyce, that she was an angel. She shares her time and energy helping the aged, infirm and troubled brothers and sisters of The Village at Westerville Retirement Center.

We have worked together for a year. She is indeed an angel. Without her dedicated work, I would still be a year away from finishing this book.

Thank you, also, to Kim Grant who assisted me in finding a publisher. She also spent many hours formatting the document to be able to submit for publishing. She has also mentioned what a privilege it was to be able to help me tell my story.

CPSIA information can be obtained at www.ICGtesting.com
Printed in the USA
LVOW082316191011

251242LV00002B/4/P

9 781448 983377